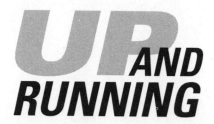

UP AND RUNNING

The Inspiring True Story of a Boy's Struggle to Survive and Triumph

Mark Patinkin

CENTER
STREET

NEW YORK   BOSTON   NASHVILLE

Center Street
Time Warner Book Group
1271 Avenue of the Americas, New York, NY 10020
Visit our website at www.twbookmark.com

The Center Street name and logo are registered trademarks
of the Time Warner Book Group.
Printed in the United States of America
First edition: September 2005
10   9   8   7   6   5   4   3   2   1

Library of Congress Cataloging-in-Publication Data

Patinkin, Mark.
    Up and running : the inspiring true story of a boy's struggle to survive and
triumph / Mark Patinkin.
        p.   cm.
    ISBN 1-931722-49-8
    1. Bateson, Andrew—Health.   2. Meningitis in children—Patients—
United States—Biography.   I. Title.
    RJ496.M45B387 2005
    362.196'82'0092—dc22   2005011917

For Ariel, Alexander,
and Zachary

Contents

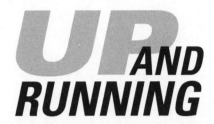

Chapter 1

"God, what's going on here?"

Less than an hour earlier, Andrew Bateson had been running outdoors with his sister and cousins. He was now shivering in bed with a temperature of 102. That's how quickly it started.

They were in Shaw's supermarket around ten o'clock the night of July 3 when Andrew said he felt sick. He said he was so tired his legs hurt. He asked his mother to carry him. Andrew had brown hair and freckles and was six years old. It was unusual for him to slow down. He was the kind of boy who would come inside for lunch with his Rollerblades on.

The family had gone to see fireworks outside Providence, where they lived. Scott and Rebecca Bateson had five kids in tow, their own two and three cousins. Afterward, everyone wanted ice cream, so they stopped by the grocery store since it was cheaper than buying cones. The cousins were sleeping over and the plan was to get all the fixings and scoop it themselves at the Batesons' house. As she waited for her husband to bring their 1990 Volvo station wagon, Rebecca pressed her cheek against Andrew's forehead and noticed how warm he was.

. . .

They gave him Tylenol and put him in their bed. The Tylenol lowered his fever, but it soon returned to 102 and remained there all night. His parents checked every hour or so. By 5 A.M., Andrew had thrown up several times. He had no energy or interest in things. He just lay there. The flu, they assumed. Around 10 A.M., something about Andrew's color bothered Rebecca. He seemed grayish. Twelve hours after her son first felt ill, she called Dr. Joseph Singer, the family's pediatrician.

The office was closed for the Fourth of July. Dr. Singer, 38, was on call, usually his busiest time. During one such stint, he returned 140 phone messages. Among the most common complaints was a child with fever and headache, perhaps fatigued and vomiting. Singer got those calls daily and assumed they were the current virus. Such kids got better on their own. He always probed anyway, looking for that one rare case that sounded like the flu but was not. Starting in medical school, Dr. Singer had been warned about this. Perhaps the biggest mistake for a pediatrician, they told him, was missing a diagnosis of bacterial meningitis.

He knew there were two forms of the disease, both potentially fatal. The more common—meningococcal meningitis—infects the membranes around the spinal fluid and brain. The other, meningococcemia, involves the blood and is more dangerous still. Once its symptoms become clear, it can be fatal in hours, despite medical treatment. Children put to bed with a slight fever have been found dead in the morning, covered with a blotchy, purplish rash. Because it mimics routine viruses, doctors cannot send every fever patient to the emergency room, or hospitals would be overrun. Pediatricians are left to poke at each call to be sure.

By the time Rebecca Bateson phoned Dr. Singer that morning of July 4, 1997, he had gotten ten similar calls: fever, vomiting, and lethargy. All proved routine. He assumed Andrew Bateson's case was the same. Rebecca described his night, then said she didn't like Andrew's color. That got Dr. Singer's attention. As meningococcemia advanced, it caused shock, slowing circulation and leaving the skin with a pallor. Instead of telling her it was a summer bug, as Rebecca had expected, Singer asked pointed questions.

Was Andrew lethargic? Unresponsive?

Well, yes.

That struck Singer, too. It was one thing for a child to feel crummy, but with meningococcemia, kids were spent, and gave little eye contact. They were basically out of it. It helped that Dr. Singer knew Rebecca. A mother's tone could be revealing. Some got nervous over every little issue; Rebecca took things in stride. Today she sounded anxious.

He asked if Andrew had a rash. Routine viruses could also cause them, but with meningococcemia, the vessels bled beneath the surface. Press most rashes, and the skin briefly turned white again. Press a hemorrhagic rash and it did not. It often began with pinpoint dots, called petechiae. If it progressed to purple welts, it meant the disease was causing septic shock, a poisoning of the blood.

No, Rebecca said, there was no sign of a rash.

The call still bothered Dr. Singer: her tone, Andrew's color. He told Rebecca she might want to bring Andrew to Hasbro Children's Hospital in Providence, at least to make sure he wasn't dehydrated.

Singer didn't mention to her that the day before, he had dealt with his first case of meningococcemia in years. A mother called about a daughter who had been vomiting and had a fever. Dr. Singer suspected the girl had a kidney infection because of a history of it. He asked the mom to bring her to the office. The girl was seven. During the exam, Singer noticed pinpoint bruising on her upper arm. He pushed the skin. The dots did not blanch white. An ambulance, he felt, might take too long. He told the mother to go to the emergency room. He was calm, but added that she should not stop at home, or any stores, since her child might have an infection needing intravenous antibiotics. He phoned the hospital to prepare them. By the time the girl got there her rash was spreading, and she was going into shock. It proved to be meningococcemia.

He could not be sure how much this influenced him when Rebecca Bateson called about Andrew. What were the odds of one pediatrician getting two such rare cases in two days?

The Batesons had planned to go to a July Fourth cookout at the home of one of Rebecca's sisters. She told Scott to go ahead with their eight-year-old daughter, Erin; she would follow after the hospital. As Rebecca got ready, Scott checked on Andrew. He was asleep in their bed, and because of the summer heat wasn't wearing a shirt. Scott noticed little spots on Andrew's chest and stomach. Why would a child with the flu have spots? He called Rebecca. To her it looked like cat scratches, but beneath the skin. She remembered what the doctor had said about a rash. A few months before, there had been an outbreak of bacterial meningitis cases in the Rhode Island city of Woonsocket. Several children had died. Rebecca recalled that she was supposed to look not just for a rash, but also a high fever, neck pain, and sensitivity to light. Andrew's fever was not above 102, and he did not have the other signs.

Still, the red marks concerned them.

"This isn't right," Scott said.

The Batesons lived on College Road in Providence, a block of fifteen modest houses and as many children. By day, the children often played outside together, as if in a 1950s television series. Rebecca went quickly across the street to ask a neighbor named Rhonda Mullen if she could watch Erin and the cousins. Rhonda came back with her and looked at Andrew. She noticed the spots. "Just go," she said. "I'll take care of the kids."

Rebecca carried Andrew to the back seat of the Volvo. To Scott, he seemed almost as if he were drugged. That got Scott's adrenaline going. He turned the ignition and just flew. He didn't exactly go through red lights, but he didn't stick around too long at them, either. He steered past anything in his way. He kept asking Rebecca how Andrew was doing. She said he wasn't moving much. When they first got in the car, Rebecca noticed that the dashboard clock said 11:11. Normally, it would take a good twenty minutes to get to the hospital. When they pulled into the emergency entrance, the clock said 11:22.

The weather was eighty degrees and fair. It occurred to Rebecca that had it been a colder day Andrew might have had a shirt on, and they could have missed the rash and been more casual about the hospital. While Rebecca carried Andrew in, Scott backed into a temporary spot next to the emergency entrance. The sign said parking was allowed there for fifteen minutes. The first chance he would have to move the car would be a considerable time after that.

Early that morning, around six-fifteen, Ted Kaiser left his home for Hasbro Hospital, where he worked as a nurse in the emergency department. He was dressed in light blue scrubs. His wife and two young children were asleep. Kaiser is six feet four inches, 220 pounds, and had played semi-pro baseball in the Cranberry League on Cape Cod, Massachusetts, until he tore up an arm. He was now thirty-six. Nursing was his third career. He began in the navy, then became a family psychologist. Fee-for-service work in the mental-health field, however, became difficult. He grew tired of calling gatekeeper agencies to beg for sessions with his kids.

This was Kaiser's fourth year in the children's ER. He had learned that kids had an interesting way of presenting themselves, such as peas up the nose and beans in the ears. You had your toddler-versus-coffee-table encounters. He also saw the not-so-pleasant cases. The ones that made him angriest were abuse situations. So did unrestrained motor vehicle accidents. Sometimes the ER would get a whole van full. He would be putting children back together and thinking all the while that this could have been prevented.

Kaiser was expecting a heavy caseload for the holiday weekend. Usually the emergency room saw more injuries—falls, cuts, and breaks—when families were relaxing at home. So far, though, it had been slow. Kaiser was assigned to the triage desk, which faced the public waiting area. A nurse always staffed it so complaints could be prioritized. A "3" meant non-urgent, a "2" urgent, and "1" meant trauma. Most of the time, 1's were bad accidents. With children, medical traumas such as a crisis illness were less frequent.

Rebecca sat her son on the waiting-room desk. Andrew leaned slackly against her shoulder. He was wearing a baseball outfit. It was given to the Batesons after a neighbor's son outgrew it. That was the kind of block College Road was; people got hand-me-downs from across the street.

Rebecca explained to Ted Kaiser how Andrew had gotten sick the previous night and still had a fever. Kaiser was supposed to fill out a brief history, but his attention was on how bad this child looked. Kaiser had a sixth sense at such times. In the same way parents can tell when their own kids were off, Kaiser believed ER staff could see it in children they were meeting for the first time.

"Let's get him started," Kaiser said, and carried Andrew into an assessment room. It had a paper-covered exam table and two scales, one for infants, another for toddlers. Getting a weight was a priority so doctors could calibrate medication.

They had not yet entered the emergency room itself, which was through a nearby pair of double doors. Scott came in from parking the car and joined them.

Kaiser knew the assessment room reminded most kids of needles and doctors' offices. To lighten the mood, he liked to say goofy things. He might look at a five-year-old and ask how he liked the sixth grade. In this case, he was moving too quickly to think about repartee. The less time this child spent out here, Kaiser thought, the better.

"Andrew?" Kaiser asked. "Can you stand, Andrew?" Scott lifted his son upright, but his legs kind of flopped. There was nothing left in him. Kaiser took Andrew's blood pressure; it was low, 60 over 40, and his heart rate fast. He knew those were signs of possible shock. Kaiser was guessing something viral, at least severe flu, probably dehydration, and then, just as he was about to do a skin assessment anyway, Rebecca told him that Andrew had a rash. Only a minute or so had gone by.

Kaiser lifted Andrew's shirt. He saw the petechiae, pinpoint red dots and scratches. Other viruses could cause this picture, but it got Kaiser's attention. He pressed some of the dots and saw that they didn't blanch. That told him they were hemorrhagic. He saw a few angrier purple spots, mostly on Andrew's trunk. They were like small welts. Those did not blanch, either. Kaiser assumed they were purpura, a sign of extreme blood infection. That was about the last thing he wanted to see on a child's skin.

Kaiser assumed this was meningococcemia. Of all diseases that came through the door, it got the most respect from the ER staff. He had seen his share of cases, many with bad outcomes. He noted one thing different about Andrew's purpura. The rash was spreading even as he watched. Kaiser had never seen meningococcemia move that fast.

"We need to treat this immediately," he told Scott and Rebecca. "We're going to take him to the trauma room." He scooped Andrew into his arms. "Let's get him back there."

He pushed a button to open the doors, then walked into the emergency unit itself, a large area with sixteen exam rooms surrounding a glassed-in nurses' station called the fishbowl.

"We need to have a doctor in the trauma room now," Kaiser called out. He also asked for the senior resident, a trauma nurse, and backup nurse.

He lay Andrew on one of the two gurneys in the trauma room. The little baseball outfit was off him now, and Rebecca was alarmed to see that the cat scratches had grown into purple blotches on his stomach, upper thighs, and neck. She wondered how such marks could spread like that. It was fortunate, she thought, that this was a holiday. Otherwise she might have taken Andrew first to the pediatrician's office.

Dr. Jim Linakis had been in the fishbowl when Kaiser called out for a doctor. The request had been calm, but when anyone used a phrase like that in the pediatric ER, it meant something. It wasn't like television, where people are shouting constantly for doctors. Since he was the attending physician, Linakis walked right over. He was forty-six, and had been associate director of the Pediatric Emergency Department for eight years. He was known as a supportive boss. Colleagues remembered him losing his temper only once, when a young intern swore at a nurse under his breath. The nurse didn't hear, but Linakis did. When he was finished responding, most who observed the exchange guessed it would be some time before the intern talked disrespectfully about a nurse again.

"He's had flu symptoms since last night," Kaiser told Linakis. "His parents said he woke up looking horrible. He's breaking out in petechiae all over."

Jim Linakis saw the rash on Andrew and immediately thought it was meningococcemia. Many doctors might have needed more time to assess, but in the previous twelve months Hasbro Children's had seen almost twenty cases, ten times normal. No one knew why, and because it was short of a mathematical epidemic, the Rhode Island Department of Health had not called for vaccination programs or other actions. Still, the Hasbro staff had become experienced with this usually rare disease.

Linakis knew it to be contagious, although minimally so. It was passed through such things as coughing, kissing, or sharing a drinking glass. But even those who got the bacteria seldom became ill. About 15 percent of the population carries meningococcus—which causes bacterial meningitis—in the throat, sometimes for months. Hosts tend to be carriers only. In a few cases, however, perhaps because of a more potent strain or an immune disturbance such as a cold, the bacteria penetrate the mucous tissues and start to spread.

Meningococcus most frequently infects the fluid and membranes around the spinal cord and brain. There are 20,000 such cases each year in the United States, with a mortality rate of 5 to 20 percent. Andrew had the more invasive form, meningococcemia, where the same bacteria multiplies in the blood. Nationally, those cases number 3,000 each year. The death rate can be well over 20 percent among patients arriving at the hospital with advancing symptoms. Most victims are younger children and babies. There are also occurrences among college students, due to close-quarter living. The most common clusters used to be in the military, but ongoing vaccination reduced that.

The bacteria, Linakis guessed, began colonizing Andrew Bateson's blood several days before, perhaps as much as a week. That was the usual incubation period, during which the host does not feel ill. Andrew's spreading rash was a sign of severe deterioration.

The next thing Rebecca knew, everybody was masking and gloving. Tubes and needles were everywhere. Linakis did not put on precautions. He realized it was bad practice, and a bad example, but at the moment, his main concern was speed. Besides, he had treated enough cases to believe that if he had not gotten it by now, he wasn't going to. He asked Andrew how he was doing.

"I'm fine," Andrew said. The response seemed lifeless. Most sick kids, even those hit by cars, were more interactive than that. Still, it was good the boy would use those words.

Dr. Linakis glanced at the mom and dad. In part, he gauged how worried he had to be by how worried the parents were. The father in particular was conveying that Andrew was much worse than the night before. Some of the spots, Linakis noticed, had grown. He wished that wasn't happening.

The previous day, the ER had received another meningococcemia patient. It was a young girl who, like Andrew, came in with petechiae. In her case, it did not turn into purpura welts. Clearly, Andrew was progressing faster. In terms of speed, Andrew was toward the top of Linakis's experience.

The worst damage of meningococcemia, Linakis knew, was caused by the reaction it triggers. Once the bacteria's toxins multiply in the blood, they ignite a destructive immunological flare-up that causes vessels to leak, organs to fail, and clotted tissues to die. In essence, at the vascular level, meningococcus drives the body into its own suicide. Some say it's akin to a match being dropped into a gasoline tank, and in fact, many who survive the first days of bacterial meningitis end up covered with the equivalent of second- and third-degree burns.

Over the speaker, Rebecca heard more people paged—"Trauma team and respiratory therapy to Trauma Room One, stat." At first Rebecca listened as if it were hospital white noise, and then it struck her: "That's us."

Mary St. Jacques was the assigned trauma nurse. She found the job stressful, and went to Florida three or four times a year to sit in the sun and decompress. The most trying part was the way children couldn't tell you what was happening with them. That also made the job challenging to her. Of her twenty-three years as a nurse, Mary had spent her last decade or so in pediatric emergency. The witching hour there tended to be around 11 A.M. As Mary put it, that's when all heck breaks loose. She noticed it was around that time when Ted Kaiser paged her. Inside, there was a boy on a gurney.

"He has the rash," Ted said. Mary understood Ted's shorthand. During the previous year, they had seen their share of it. The rash alarmed her. It was spreading; the child was going septic before her eyes.

"Andrew," she said, "my name's Mary. I'm one of the nurses. I'm going to take care of you."

The temperature in the trauma room was over eighty degrees, kept that way because patients there were often in shock. The room's cabinets were filled with such things as vascular cut-down kits for the opening of the chest, a kit for delivering babies, and a neuro kit capable of boring a hole through the skull to relieve cranial pressure. A respiratory cart had endotracheal tubes for intubation. There were resuscitative drugs and a "code cart" equipped with epinephrine and atropine to restart a stopped heart. Behind Andrew's gurney, there was a suction canister, for either the removal of excess blood or the decompression of the stomach. There were two defibrillators, the second a backup in case the first malfunctioned. The staff was required to retest both during each shift and restock whatever else had been used. They understood there would be little time for that when the next patient came in.

Dr. Jim Linakis did not encourage a lot of shouting when he was attending a trauma. He preferred one leader in the room. That way, nurses knew who was giving instructions and could hear clearly. When treating Andrew, he didn't have to say much. The staff moved quickly, having done this more than once in the past year.

Mary told Andrew she was going to put him on the monitor. "It doesn't hurt," she said. "I'm going to give your arm a hug with a balloon to take your blood pressure." He did not resist. His arm remained limp. Someone put stickers on Andrew's chest. The Spacelabs monitor began to display cardiac and respiratory rates. They put a Pulseox clip on his finger that shined an infrared beam through the capillary beds, gauging blood-oxygen saturation. Beneath his chin, they attached a mask that sent up a mist of oxygen through sterile water.

Mary prepared an intravenous line. With a child as sick as Andrew you needed several two-way ports; in for medications, out for bloodwork. She used a yellow rubber tube for a tourniquet on his arm, then probed for a good vein inside his elbow. Once in, she announced she had a line, right "antecube," twenty-two gauge. Ted Kaiser worked to start an additional line, inserting a large-bore needle. He was aware of the parents as he did this. People were ambivalent about their kids being stuck. He threaded an IV catheter tube through the needle and anchored it. From those lines they would first draw blood, then infuse Andrew with antibiotics and fluids.

Scott Bateson saw one needle put into his son's wrist, another into his ankle; Andrew did not flinch or cry. The parents had to stay out of everyone's way since the staff was moving urgently. So far, only minutes had gone by since Andrew was brought into trauma.

Ted Kaiser tried not to dwell on how improbable it was that a child with so advanced a case of meningococcemia would survive. It was like in baseball: If you thought about throwing balls, you'd throw balls. Better to think about strikes. Briefly, he tried such a focus, but there really wasn't much time to get into that.

A nurse asked what kind of bloods Linakis wanted. "Let's get a CBC with diff, sed rate, blood culture, set of electrolytes, co-ags, DIC screen," he said. He asked for a clot sent to the blood bank so they could match Andrew's type. He asked for PT, PTT, and fibrin splits, indirect ways of confirming meningococcemia. A lumbar puncture would have given Linakis a more precise determination: You tapped the spine for cerebrospinal fluid and tested it for signs of infection. They began to talk about it. Someone asked if they should do it down here in the ER or wait until he got up to intensive care.

Linakis decided Andrew wasn't stable enough to turn him on his side, bunch him into a ball, and push a needle near his cord. Besides, Linakis didn't need a test to tell him how to proceed. He knew what he was looking at. The question wasn't what was going on with the patient, it was whether they could stop it.

Linakis pictured what was happening inside Andrew's body. Upon sensing the spread of bacteria, Andrew's immune system would have sent in white blood cells. Those cells would release packages of protective enzymes that would degranulate and cover the invaders. Meningococcus, however, had triggered Andrew's immune system to overreact, sending an irrational number of white cells into the fight, perhaps 10,000 against each invader when a few would have done. Andrew's body had released swarms of other immune agents as well, including cytokines and other proteins. It had flooded his body with interleukins and platelets. At such illogical volume, these protectors became toxic to the very host they were supposed to guard. The effect, internally, was akin to aiming a blowtorch at a mosquito upon the neck.

"Let's draw up a hundred per kilo of ceftriaxone," Linakis said. "We could go ahead and push that as soon as it's ready." Ceftriaxone was the strongest antibiotic they had. They gave Andrew the maximum amount. They pushed it through several intravenous lines at once.

"Is the antibiotic in yet?"

"Yes, most of it."

Linakis knew ceftriaxone worked quickly. Soon the bacteria in Andrew would begin to die. One thing doctors knew how to do was kill meningococcus; it isn't a robust organism. Still, it by now had begun its damage, releasing millions of endotoxins into Andrew's blood. As each meningococcal bacterium fell apart due to the antibiotic, it released still more poisonous molecules, accelerating the inflammatory cascade that was causing Andrew's body to turn on itself.

It seemed wherever Rebecca stood, a nurse bumped into her. Every so often, they would give words of encouragement.

"Think positive," one said. "A girl came in yesterday and is doing better today."

The assurance startled Rebecca. She thought: *Why* wouldn't *you recover from this?*

The medical people kept asking Andrew how he was doing. He would murmur, "All right." But he seemed far away.

Linakis continued to picture Andrew's physiological breakdown. When the body first sensed unwanted bacteria, the normal reaction was for vessels to dilate, allowing antibodies to come inside and attack the invader cells. Meningococcus, however, by triggering too many antibodies, caused Andrew's vessels to overdilate, becoming dangerously porous. Plasma was now leaking from his veins and arteries at a speed causing him to bleed internally. Andrew's blood pressure continued to decline. As it did, his ability to carry oxygen to his organs and tissues became more and more compromised.

"Let's give him some fluid," Linakis said. He asked for twenty cubic centimeters per kilo of normal saline. Ted Kaiser grabbed a one-liter bag kept in a heater at body temperature. He hung it on an IV pole. They routed the saline through an additional warmer before it entered Andrew's body.

It was common enough for Linakis to see shock in an emergency room. Usually it was the result of dehydration or blood loss, perhaps from a car accident. Put simply, a patient's tank got low. You wouldn't use a powerful medication like dopamine for that; you just needed to refill the tank by replacing volume. Once doctors infused a bag of fluid or blood, it usually did the job. The shock caused by meningococcemia was different. It was called septic shock, and made blood vessels so leaky that almost as quickly as doctors poured volume in, it seeped out again. Nurse Mary St. Jacques knew children could hold blood pressure and heart rate longer than adults, having a mechanism to compensate for shock. On the other hand, once children's pressure began to drop hard, they were more prone to crash.

As Andrew slipped deeper into shock, his body pulled its diminished blood supply to his heart and brain. In so doing, it shut down flow to the extremities. The skin there took on an increasingly gray cast.

Dr. Linakis felt Andrew's legs. Although the room was over eighty degrees and Andrew's temperature 102, his legs were cold to the touch. Linakis pressed Andrew's thumbnail until it turned white. Normally, it would quickly pink up again. Now it took four or five seconds to do so. It was the same when they pressed elsewhere on his skin, particularly the legs.

"His perfusion stinks," Linakis said. He guessed it was more than just circulatory collapse. The heart, hampered by the inflammatory reaction, was not working efficiently. That was predictable. Judging by Andrew's mental state, Linakis figured his brain wasn't well oxygenated either. The body was also pulling blood from organs that used a lot of it, such as the kidneys, putting those in jeopardy as well.

Linakis asked for an additional twenty cc's per kilo of normal saline. It was likely that those fluids would leak from Andrew's vessels too. So far, Linakis had given Andrew about a half liter, equivalent to one-quarter of his total blood volume, and he doubted it would be enough. He would have to pour in more, which could lead to other problems. Because kidney failure was all but certain, Andrew's body would be unable to expel the excess fluid. It would stay in him, filling the spaces between his organs and under his skin. He would begin to bloat, the swelling making it hard for him to breathe. In the worst case, fluid would start seeping into Andrew's lungs.

"What do you think about starting dopamine?" Linakis asked those around him.

At the right dose, dopamine might tighten Andrew's vessels, slowing leakage and boosting blood pressure. Just as important, it would make his heart beat harder, squeezing blood to places that could use some, like his kidneys.

But dopamine was serious medication. You did not want to administer it to a child unless necessary. "His BP's pretty stable," someone answered. "Why do you want to start it?"

Linakis wondered if yesterday's meningococcemia case fed into the hesitancy. That girl had never progressed to a crisis. Mightn't Andrew stabilize too? Then Linakis considered how different the two were. Already Andrew was sicker than the young girl ever got.

"Do you believe we had two of these in a row?" someone said.

"Hopefully," said Linakis, "this one will do as well as the munchkin yesterday, but that's not what he's showing us right now."

Linakis checked the monitor for Andrew's last several blood pressures. He disagreed that they were stable. They were erratic, and going in the wrong direction.

"I'm concerned he's going to crash and burn," Linakis said. He instructed a nurse to start administering dopamine. He saw the rash continue to spread. He almost said "God, what's going on here?" but he was mindful of the parents.

Linakis found it startling to see a meningococcemia patient go septic after having come into the hospital so early. Staffers began calling out Andrew's rates. His blood pressure had been boosted back to 109 over 64 by the dopamine but was falling again. His oxygen levels were falling too, toward 80 percent. Normal saturation—sats—was 100 percent, or close to it. Anything below the high 80s was problematic. Andrew's body wasn't getting much oxygen.

Someone said, "Purpura is getting progressively worse." The spots on Andrew's abdomen and legs were turning into welts. Same with his arms. Linakis considered the progression scary.

"We have any blood results back?"

No. It had been only minutes since a certified nursing assistant had taken them to the lab. To Linakis it seemed much longer.

Jim Linakis thought he should talk to the Batesons. They did not yet know how grave their child's condition was.

"May I speak to you?"

Rebecca wanted to stay with Andrew. Scott followed the doctor to a nearby family room. "I just want to let you know what I think is going on in Andrew," Linakis said. "Of course, to be certain about this, we have to get cultures back from the blood test. But what I'm pretty sure Andrew has is meningococcemia."

Scott's head went right to meningitis. He had seen newspaper stories and remembered it as a serious sickness. Linakis wanted to be reassuring, but had learned that when parents are encouraged and things then go badly, it's more devastating.

"This disease is very dangerous," Linakis told Scott. "I can't be really sure. I can't guarantee you that Andrew will survive."

Scott asked how that was possible.

"Meningococcemia," Linakis said, "is very rapid." He told Scott that by now they had probably destroyed the bacteria that had caused Andrew to fall ill. But all the toxins, the by-products of the bacteria, were still in his body. That was causing the damage.

Scott didn't understand this. If the disease itself had been killed, why would Andrew be in danger of not surviving?

"What Andrew is going through from this point on," Linakis said, "is his body now has to fight off all these toxins." How that would unfold, he told Scott, was uncertain.

"Time is what saves the person," Linakis added. "It's the whole thing, getting the patient to the hospital quickly. And you did," he told Scott. Then Linakis said he needed to get back with Andrew.

Scott returned to the trauma room. He told Rebecca that Andrew had a bad form of meningitis. He could die from it. Scott broke down a little, and so did she, but only briefly, because Andrew was conscious enough to be aware of their reactions. Scott asked Andrew how he was doing. He felt if he could just get his son to stay awake and respond, things would be okay.

Andrew would murmur "All right," but only barely.

Rebecca asked a nurse if her son was going to die.

"Think positively," the nurse said. Others repeated similar words. When Rebecca looked at their eyes, she did not see optimism.

One of Rebecca's sisters, Deb Powers, worked in nuclear medicine at a nearby hospital. They knew she would be getting ready for the family's July Fourth gathering. Scott dialed her number on his cell phone.

"Deb," Scott said. "Could you please come to Hasbro? Andrew's really sick. I don't know what's going on, but he may not survive. They said it's meningitis."

Even as plasma continued to leak inside Andrew, Linakis knew another part of his system was causing perhaps greater problems. His clotting mechanisms were out of control. When a normal immune system senses a nick or tear in a blood vessel, it sends platelets to clot it off. Andrew's system had overreacted, perceiving every part of his leaking vessels as nicks in need of repair. In response, his body had released an unhealthy flood of platelets. They formed tiny clots, which began to flow like a black snowstorm through his vessels. Some of the clots snagged here and there. Most flowed until they reached the endpoint capillaries, which fed oxygen to the tissues. There, like flecks of tar, the clots began to choke entire capillary beds, cutting off patches of his body. That was what had first caused the petechiae and then the purpura. By now Andrew had so many such welts his skin resembled a ruined landscape.

Linakis did not know how deep the purpura damage would go. In severe cases of patients who survived it reached to bone, and skin grafts were required. Some spots, Ted Kaiser noticed, were appearing on Andrew's face. Dr. Linakis kept feeling Andrew's legs and hands. They were getting colder. That told him clots were obstructing the vessels to his limbs. In addition, Andrew's body was pulling his blood to his core organs. Andrew's feet and hands, being endpoints, were the first to be cut off. If this process was not reversed, Linakis knew, the extremities could die.

Mary St. Jacques noticed Rebecca's sister, Deb Powers, outside the trauma-room doors. The two happened to be friends. Mary stepped away to talk to her. She saw no point in trying to hide what was happening around another hospital person.

"Deb, he's real sick. We're worried about him." Deb Powers understood what that was code for. The faces of the staffers gave the same message whenever the doors opened.

. . .

The monitors told Linakis that Andrew's air exchange was adequate, enough oxygen in and carbon dioxide out, but he questioned how long it would remain so. Linakis thought Andrew's body needed more help. Could they lighten the load by breathing for him? Sooner or later, Linakis guessed, Andrew would have to be tubed.

"Do you think we'll do him any favor by intubating him?" he asked.

"Well," someone answered, "he seems to be protecting his airway pretty well right now."

Linakis nodded. "Why don't we get him up to the unit and see how he does there."

The function of the emergency room was to stabilize patients for intensive care. Linakis thought this work was close to finished. The antibiotics were in, and they had decided against a ventilator. A bit less than an hour had gone by since Andrew arrived.

"Is the unit ready to take him?"

"Yes," Mary St. Jacques said.

Linakis told everyone, "Let's get him going."

It took a bit of doing to transfer all of Andrew's support equipment to the gurney. They put his wires into a portable monitor and set it next to him. They put the oxygen underneath, and hung IV pumps on attached poles. A nurse and technician began pushing the gurney while Dr. Linakis walked alongside. Because of the sensitivity of Andrew's state, they moved slowly. Even small jostling could impact him. It made Linakis anxious. If Andrew went downhill, you could only do so much for him in transit. Andrew didn't move or cry.

Deb Powers walked with them. The children's nickname for Deb was "Aunt Love." She called her nieces and nephews that word—"C'mon, love"—and it caught on. Andrew used it now. "Aunt Love," he said, "can you make me better?"

"Pal, I'll do my best."

. . .

Mary St. Jacques wheeled Andrew to the back elevators. Outside a nearby window there was a sculpture of porpoises leaping from a flat roof. Mary took out her override key and inserted it, instructing the elevator to come directly.

Scott looked down at his son. It was hard to grasp how the spots could have gotten so much bigger. The elevator doors closed. Scott looked at the wall. It was covered with reflective metal bumps that were somewhat hypnotizing. His gaze stayed there and he was lost in his thoughts.

No one talked while they rode up. It had often been Ted Kaiser's experience that this was where you could hear parents pray, even if they were doing it silently.

The trip from the ER to the ICU was five minutes, and in that time Andrew's rash grew further. Linakis had never seen that before. He thought to himself, *God, he's got a lot of purpura.* Andrew arrived at the pediatric intensive care unit around 12:15 P.M. His condition was critical and deteriorating. The PICU had been kept informed by phone, but it was protocol to give a report anyway, nurse-to-nurse.

"This is Andrew," said Mary St. Jacques. "Six-year-old with possible meningococcemia . . ."

Linakis escorted the parents to a waiting room and let them know the PICU needed a half hour to get Andrew set up. Rebecca and Scott asked if there was something more they could have done to prevent this. He told them there was nothing. They had gotten him in as quickly as any rational parent could. As Linakis phrased it, this was just a bad disease that came on faster than gangbusters.

Mary was in the room as Andrew was placed into his new bed. She did not stay long since there were a lot of people working in there. As she was leaving, she said a small prayer. Inside, the PICU nurses continued the resuscitation even as they settled him in.

Scott looked through the window of Andrew's room. It faced the nurses' station, standard in the ICU, so patients could be watched steadily. They were hooking so many lines and machines to his son that Scott could not keep track.

At last the parents were allowed to go in. Andrew had been placed in an isolation room. To get inside, Scott and Rebecca first had to enter an anteroom and put on gowns, gloves, and masks. Andrew was still awake. He seemed distant. His body had swelled from all the fluids.

"Mom," he said, "I'm so thirsty."

Rebecca asked if she could give him some ice chips.

A nurse told her it wasn't possible.

At least touch a wet cloth against his lips?

"I'm sorry," the nurse said, "but you can't."

Mary St. Jacques went back to the trauma room to clean up. She scrubbed down the table, washed the pumps, returned the monitor to position. She replaced used equipment and medications. When she was done, she asked the others if they could cover for her. She needed five minutes. She went to the break room, where they kept coffee. Once there, while alone, she fell apart for a few seconds.

Jim Linakis returned to his desk in the fishbowl. By then, the department had backed up. Everyone wanted his attention. He had only a minute or so. He lifted the phone and dialed home. His wife, Gloria, answered.

"We just had this really tough case," he told her. "This incredibly sick kid. I don't know if he's going to live."

Linakis had been doing this work for fifteen years, but at such times still pictured his own children. He and his wife had five, ages two to fourteen.

"How's everybody doing?" he asked.

His wife told him everyone was fine. He told her he had to get back to work.

Five hours later, around 6 P.M., Linakis signed out of the ER. He took the back elevator to the PICU. Dr. Monica Kleinman was at the central desk when he got there. She was the attending that night. Linakis considered her one of the best doctors he knew. Andrew was now her patient.

"How's he doing?" he asked.

She said Linakis was welcome to go in and see him. He gowned up. The parents were both there. Linakis could barely believe how much Andrew had declined. His body was so covered with purpura it appeared spackled with tar. Linakis had never seen a meningococcemia patient in such extreme condition. When he first brought Andrew into the PICU, Linakis thought he had a chance at surviving, although with deficits. He no longer believed that.

Ted Kaiser worked a double that day, so it was evening before he got off. Around 8 P.M., he went upstairs to see Andrew. Several nurses were around him, making constant adjustments. Because of their resilience, sick children tend to look better than sick adults. Andrew was not that way. He was puffy and blown up like a balloon. Most of his skin was blackish brown, as if from burns. It was one of the worst presentations Kaiser had seen, including car accidents. Parents, he knew, look carefully at the reaction of the providers, so he worked to maintain his composure.

Mary St. Jacques believed it was best not to get attached to every kid who came through, but there was something about Andrew. Despite being such a sick little guy, he had hung in there. Before leaving for home, Mary went upstairs to the PICU. She approached the attending physician, Dr. Monica Kleinman. She usually didn't address doctors by their first names, but she had known Kleinman for years.

"Monica," she said, "is he going to make it?"

"He's real sick," Kleinman said. "I don't know if he'll make it through the night."

That evening, Mary's sister was expecting her for a cookout. Mary called and explained about the boy she had treated. She said she wasn't up to going out.

"Why don't you?" her sister said. "You'll feel better."

Mary apologized. She knew it was hard for people not in the medical field to understand. She sat by herself in her backyard and sent up another prayer.

The activity around Andrew was nonstop. Scott and Rebecca sat silently next to their son. Something got Scott thinking about Andrew's bicycle. It was shaped like a Harley-Davidson motorcycle. Andrew had seen it in a toy store and for weeks talked of little else. It was waiting for him under the tree Christmas morning. It turned out to be too much bike for him. He continued to try riding it every so often anyway. He couldn't wait to grow into it.

Chapter 2

"You don't have a choice . . ."

D r. Monica Kleinman called her staff around the nurses' station. That week, she was the doctor in charge of Hasbro's intensive care unit. She told them they had a likely meningococcemia case, a six-year-old boy.

"This youngster is going to be quite unstable," she said. "He's going to need a lot of intervention quickly." She could almost hear people take a breath when she mentioned meningococcemia.

Dr. Kleinman said they would likely get the new admission in about a half hour. At the time, Andrew was still being worked on in the trauma room downstairs. Kleinman phoned Jim Linakis, the ER attending.

"Jim, I hear you have a patient for me. Where are things at?"

"This is pretty impressive," he told her. "He's evolving purpura by the minute."

Although several things could have caused a spreading hemorrhagic rash, the first five on Dr. Kleinman's list were meningococcemia.

"He's going to be a sick one," said Linakis.

Dr. Kleinman phoned her husband, Gary. On a normal July Fourth she could sometimes get lucky and be home by 1 P.M. That seemed improbable. "I'm going to be here for the foreseeable future," she said. Gary asked her to keep him posted.

She had left home before 7 A.M. in her Subaru Outback, stopping to buy pastries for the unit. While in training, she had been struck by some attendings who would bring doughnuts for everyone. It was a morale booster to have a boss treat you that way.

She tried to keep her own breakfast something healthy, like Raisin Bran, since she never knew when she might eat next. Lately she had been skipping it, having felt too ill. The nausea had been so nonstop she decided morning sickness was the wrong label; it was more like twenty-four-hour-a-day sickness. She knew of no doctor tricks to stop it. A friend advised her to have at least something in her stomach, so she tried Saltines, which worked only a little. She and Gary had been married eleven years, and this would be their first. Dr. Kleinman had been a coffee drinker, but now even the smell of it made her queasy. The lack of caffeine left her more tired than usual. At 11:30, four and a half hours into her workday, the ER had called her about Andrew Bateson.

"We need to get an art line set up, and a central line kit," Dr. Kleinman told her staff. "We should also have an epi drip." She requested fluids to infuse Andrew. The nurses organized normal saline and albumin. Kleinman had asked the ER if he had been intubated. Not so far. That, she thought, could be likely after the boy got to her. When meningococcemia was advancing, most children needed ventilator support. Kleinman had her team ready the medications for it. She expected this to be an ongoing resuscitation—overseeing the airway, starting IVs, pushing volume, constant bedside management at a pace more typical of emergency trauma.

The nurses worked quickly to prepare the room, stacking supplies behind the power column at the head of the bed. They knew they would need them nearby. The nurses had experience with this disease. They didn't have to wait to be asked to do every little thing.

. . .

The PICU charge nurse told Michele Rozenberg she would be assigned to the new admission. Michele had worked in the ICU sixteen years. Meningococcemia was the last thing she wanted to hear a patient was coming upstairs with. The children swelled to the point of distortion, their skin so taut their eyes could not open. The rash made them look like burn victims. It was quite heartbreaking.

Andrew soon arrived on a rolling gurney. He had an oxygen mask on his face. The ER staffers around him were gowned and gloved. They weren't exactly running with him, but they were moving quickly.

They wheeled Andrew into 228, an isolation room, closing all the doors. As long as he was there, everyone had to enter through an anteroom, washing hands and gowning up. Room circulation was set for negative pressure, isolating air drawn in and venting it outside the hospital. Such a precaution was typical of more contagious diseases like tuberculosis, but with meningococcemia, Dr. Kleinman preferred to be careful.

Kleinman walked into the room. Andrew looked extremely sick, but was awake and glancing around. She told him her name and asked how he was feeling. He answered in an impassive voice: "Fine." Kleinman took down his johnny to look at his chest. She had to keep herself from reacting. His torso was covered with dark blotches. The speed of this progression was unsettling.

Dr. Kleinman listened to Andrew's lungs, then pressed on the skin of his legs to check circulation. The color came back slowly. His hands and feet were cool, the pulses weak. When she looked back at his chest, some of the blotches were bigger. She thought to herself, *My God*. What normally took hours was taking minutes. His clotting mechanisms had gone haywire. The resulting welts, Kleinman knew, would end up like third-degree burns.

Ideally, thought Kleinman, you took parents aside early to prepare them, but in this case there was too much to do. She instructed the two residents to place an arterial line. They inserted a needle on the underside of Andrew's wrist. They now had constant blood-pressure readings. The line also let them draw blood samples for the lab.

Dr. Kleinman was surprised that Andrew was still responsive. Usually in septic shock of this severity, a child first grew anxious, then declined and became unconscious. Andrew was able to answer questions. It impressed her that he was strong enough to do so. Personality, Kleinman thought, could be a factor in overcoming illness.

"How are you feeling now, Andrew?"

"I'm fine."

She asked the nurses to keep up the antibiotics started in the ER— ceftriaxone, 1,000 milligrams. She assumed the meningococcus had been killed with the first dose; it's an almost feeble organism in the face of antibiotics. But she wanted to be sure.

At the same time, it was no longer the bacteria itself that concerned Kleinman, but the inflammatory reaction it had triggered.

Dr. Kleinman checked the monitor. Despite fluids and dopamine, Andrew's pressure remained low, 80 over 30. The septic shock, she assumed, had left his blood vessels dilated and floppy. Fluid was leaking out of them into his tissues. Outwardly he appeared bloated, but inside, his veins and arteries were half empty. He needed more volume.

"Let's give twenty cc's per kilo of albumin," Dr. Kleinman said. By now, he had plenty of IVs, but Kleinman didn't think they were big enough to support a child with collapsing pressure.

"Please see if you could get a femoral line set up," she told the residents. "In the interim, I'm going to talk to the parents." It had been twenty minutes since Andrew had arrived at the ICU.

A lot was going to happen in a short time, and Dr. Kleinman needed to prepare the mom and dad. She also wanted them to know who was taking care of their child. Kleinman believed parents were almost as important as medicine. The more they were involved, the better kids did. Sometimes parents showed anger, taking it out on the PICU staff. Dr. Kleinman understood. God knows how she would behave were it her child. The important thing was to see them involved.

The family waiting room was just outside the unit's double doors. The parents were sitting on a couch. Mom had her head in her hands, the father an arm around her. Kleinman told Scott and Rebecca she would be their son's doctor. She asked what their understanding was of his condition.

The father had trouble pronouncing it. Meninge . . . something. That's all they had absorbed.

"Andrew," Kleinman said, "is a very sick little boy. He has a serious infection. We're going to have to move quickly to take care of him over the next several hours. His condition is very critical and we are doing everything we can for him. But I suspect he's going to get worse."

Rebecca said they were supposed to go on vacation in two days. Did Dr. Kleinman think that would happen? Even as Rebecca asked that, she was aware it was an absurd question, but she found this hard to comprehend.

Kleinman did not feel a vacation was possible. She was confident that Andrew had bacterial meningitis, and named the specific form of it.

Meningo-something, Scott heard her say; that big long word again.

"At the moment," Kleinman said, "we're starting IVs that will help us monitor him and take care of him."

How did Andrew get it?

It was hard to catch, Kleinman said, but you got it through close contact with carriers. About 15 percent of the population had the bug in their throats but remained immune. No one knew for sure why it got through with some kids.

Antibiotics, she said, had by now likely killed the bacteria in Andrew, but the worst phase of the disease was still ahead of them.

Scott didn't understand that. If the disease was neutralized, shouldn't Andrew improve?

Kleinman explained the bacteria had triggered a toxic reaction that was breaking down the organs of Andrew's body. It was as if his system had been poisoned. He would likely have major organ failure.

Scott said, "There's nothing you can do to stop this?"

"There's really nothing," said Dr. Kleinman. The toxins were in his tissues. His body was in severe inflammatory response, which meant massive clotting and the internal leaking of fluids. "We can keep his heart pumping, and help him to breathe. We can't stop this part of it."

"He's not going to die," Rebecca said, "is he?"

"I'll try my very, very best," Kleinman said, "but he's a very sick little boy, and you have to prepare yourself for that possibility."

Rebecca said, "You can't let him die. He can't die. You can't."

"We're going to do everything we can to make sure he doesn't. We'll be with him all the time. But some children with this infection don't survive."

Rebecca's sister Deb was in the room. She watched Kleinman's face, which was grave. Deb worked in a hospital and recognized the expression.

Kleinman said she was quite certain Andrew would need a ventilator to support his breathing, perhaps within the next hour.

The parents were pretty shell-shocked. Dr. Kleinman was concerned about how much they had heard. Then she excused herself. She needed to go back to Andrew. She felt as if she had dropped a bomb and left.

Neither parent spoke for a while. They were trying to comprehend all that had been said.

"But I was just talking to him," Rebecca said.

When Kleinman got back to Andrew's bedside, his welts had expanded. It alarmed her. *Okay,* she thought, *I see how this one's going to be.* Very swift. Very aggressive.

Andrew's mental status had also changed. He was confused. He tossed his head from side to side. His breathing, fast before, had become labored. He was not getting enough oxygen, and acid had built up in his bloodstream. His body's way of trying to get rid of it was to hyperventilate, but that used up more oxygen, building still more acid. Kleinman worried that he could vomit and inhale. It was critical to keep his airway open.

"He's going to go downhill fast," she said to her team. It was time to put him on a ventilator. She had expected intubation to be farther down the road. This was the quickest she had seen a meningococcemia victim deteriorate.

Kleinman wanted Scott and Rebecca to see their son a last time without the tube in his mouth. She also wanted Andrew to know they were there before they put him under. Instead of dispatching a nurse to get the parents, she went herself. She found them on the same waiting-room couch.

"As I thought might happen," Kleinman told them, "Andrew is getting sicker. I told you before that I thought we were going to have to put him on a ventilator. It's time to do that."

Neither parent spoke.

"He's still holding his own," Dr. Kleinman said. "But he's getting uncomfortable. He's having a hard time breathing." She wanted to intubate him before it became a crisis.

A crisis?

"This is an extremely aggressive infection," she explained. "Eventually, his kidneys may fail, his heart may fail. We're going to try to stay one step ahead of that, but these are things we have to face." With meningococcemia, she said, as soon as you got over one hurdle, there was something else.

Andrew would be sedated, she explained, and remain so as long as he was on the machine. Basically, he would be in an induced coma. It would probably last weeks. The way Rebecca understood it, Andrew's body was going to go through such torment he would be likelier to fail were he aware of it.

Rebecca asked again: "But he's not going to die, is he?"

"When I can look at you in the eye and tell you he won't die, I will do that," Dr. Kleinman said.

She advised the parents to go say their good-byes and tell Andrew they would see him later.

Rebecca's sisters noticed that she had begun to shake physically, as if chilled. "I didn't think she meant that," Rebecca said of the plan to ventilate. "I thought she was just preparing us for the worst."

Scott had his arm around Rebecca. At other times, he took her hand. They were kind of holding on to each other.

It had been a half hour since the Batesons had last seen their son. He was now even more covered in purple bruises. To Rebecca he seemed so little in that bed, and the tubes going into him so large. Andrew asked if he could go home. He was more lucid than Dr. Kleinman expected.

"You're going to spend the night in the hospital with us," Dr. Kleinman said.

Rebecca told Andrew he was very sick, and the doctor would be helping him. "We're going to give you a little snoozy," Dr. Kleinman said, "and when you wake up, you'll feel so much better."

"Okay," Andrew said.

She told him Mom and Dad would be right there when he woke. Both parents said they loved him, and that the doctors would make him better.

"Okay," Andrew said again.

Kleinman advised they not stay for the intubation. It wasn't like on television dramas, where patients were tubed almost casually every few minutes. The pushing of the metal blade into the mouth was unnerving. There was always tension in the room.

"It's time for us to go ahead and take care of this procedure," Kleinman said. "I'll come and get you in the family room as soon as we're done."

As the Batesons walked back into the corridor, Rebecca broke down a little, and Scott did, too. He hoped Andrew understood they would remain by him. Scott wondered if this would be the last time he would talk to his son.

. . .

"Okay," Kleinman said to the team, "I want atropine .4 milligrams, ketamine 40 milligrams, and 20 milligrams of sux." The atropine was to protect Andrew from bradycardia, a slowing of the heart triggered by the metal blade against the vagus nerve in the throat. The ketamine was a sedative, the sux—succinylcholine—a paralytic. She chose to let one of her residents do the insertion so Kleinman could watch the monitors and direct things.

"We're going to do a rapid sequence," said Kleinman. Ideally, she hoped, they would push the meds one after another, hold cricoid pressure, and intubate without having to give breaths with a bag. Once they pushed the medications, Andrew's diaphragm would be paralyzed and there was no turning back. To prepare for the interval where he wouldn't be breathing, they had spent the last few minutes hyperoxygenating him. Dr. Kleinman looked at the monitors to make sure oxygen saturation was holding.

"Everybody ready?" They all had white surgical masks on. Kleinman glanced at their eyes. She nodded at Michele Rozenberg.

"Michele, atropine." Michele pushed the atropine into an IV port.

"Ketamine." Michele pushed that.

"Sux." She pushed the succinylcholine.

Andrew's heart rate and blood pressure held. Perhaps this said something hopeful about this child, perhaps it was luck. Kleinman watched the clock for thirty seconds to let the meds take effect. Except for machinery noises, the room was quiet. Everyone kept their eyes on Kleinman, as they needed to be on the same page. She watched Andrew's body. As planned, he had stopped breathing.

In cases of shock, where circulation slows, medications take longer to work. So Kleinman waited fifteen seconds more. It was important that he was completely paralyzed. Those seconds were another reason it was best the parents were out of the room. Andrew lay so still as to appear dead.

"Okay, put the tube in."

A resident placed the laryngoscope into Andrew's mouth to lift his tongue and jaw. Kleinman put two fingers near his Adam's apple, compressing the esophagus between the tracheal cartilage and his vertebrae to keep him from regurgitating.

"What do you see?" she asked the resident.

Andrew's vocal cords had relaxed.

"Go ahead and put in the tube."

The resident inserted the endotracheal tube. Kleinman felt it go past her fingers, stopping a few centimeters below, where the lungs branched. A respiratory therapist attached an ambu bag to the end of the tube and squeezed it, giving Andrew air for the first time in almost a minute. A nurse had a stethoscope on his chest.

"Breath sounds," she affirmed, "both sides."

They attached a carbon dioxide detector to the end of the tube to make sure it hadn't slipped into the wrong canal. A strip on the detector went from purple to yellow. They were in.

Kleinman let go of Andrew's throat. They taped the tube against Andrew's mouth while the therapist squeezed the bag. Then they attached the tube to the ventilator.

"Thanks, everyone," said Dr. Kleinman. "That was by the book."

Kleinman asked the residents to work with the respiratory therapist on ventilator settings. Then she left to tell the parents Andrew had tolerated the procedure well. They could be with their son now. The two went to his bedside.

It felt like a different room to Rebecca and Scott. Andrew was unconscious, the respirator breathing for him. There were intravenous poles all over. Two dozen lines wound across the floor like spaghetti. Tubes from IV bags dovetailed into central lines attached to pumps, and, in turn, to Andrew. There were beeps and buzzes from monitors. If an IV got low, an alarm went off. He lay on a sophisticated air mattress fed with a constant flow. It could be adjusted for warmth or coolness to support his temperature. The mattress made a low humming noise.

The space felt busy. Along with Kleinman, at least two nurses were constantly in the room, sometimes more. Rebecca and Scott tried to understand the monitors. They listened to exchanges and looked closely at Dr. Kleinman's eyes as she studied the data. One of the nurses told them that five years ago, there was almost no survival rate for a case of meningococcemia as severe as Andrew's. Now, because of all of this, there was at least a chance.

Rebecca grew up in the blue-collar town of West Warwick, Rhode Island, the youngest of four daughters. Her father was a newspaper circulation director, her mother in sales with Filene's. After Rhode Island College, Rebecca got into retail herself, working also in Filene's, then Casual Corner and Hit-or-Miss. She lived with her folks.

Scott was one of five children raised in another small, blue-collar city, East Providence. His father was an electronics technician, his mother a clerical worker at Amica Insurance. He graduated from East Providence High School in 1970 and went to work, first in warehouse inventory, then as a printer. On the side, he got a degree in chemical technology at the Community College of Rhode Island.

The two met at an ice skating class. Rebecca was twenty-three and Scott ten years older. Six weeks later, Scott took her to a nice restaurant and had the waitress bring a ring on a tray with a rose and champagne. Rebecca said yes, but told Scott he first needed to speak to her father; that was how it was done in the Dugdale home. Fred Dugdale heard Scott out, then said that given the short courtship, he wouldn't put deposits on a band or hall yet, in case the two changed their minds.

They were married ten months later, May 12, 1985. Scott's parents owned a two-family. He and Rebecca moved into the upstairs apartment. After two years, they bought a small house on College Road in Providence, a block from the gates of Providence College. Erin was born in October of 1988, Andrew in February of 1991. Scott was now working in quality control for a printer. Rebecca did day care out of her home for neighborhood kids, and would later become a secretary at St. Pius, the family's church.

The speed at which the rash spread was incredible to Scott. You could leave the room for ten minutes and the welts got bigger. Some had begun to merge together, especially on Andrew's face. It was as if you could see the disease growing on him. Kleinman explained that it was caused by clotting blood, laced with toxins, that had leaked through Andrew's blood vessels.

Rebecca's sisters looked through the window from the adjoining isolation room. Andrew's face appeared almost black. Deb Powers, the older sister, found him barely recognizable except for his hair. To Jennifer Lusignon, it looked like he had been in a fire. The welts were everywhere. Their color had gone from red to purple to black. His torso was half covered.

Rebecca asked, "When is it going to stop?"

Some cases, said Dr. Kleinman, were more extreme than others. They could not predict how far this would go. Dr. Kleinman took Polaroid photographs of Andrew. She explained that this was both for his medical records and possible reconstruction.

"You mean," said Rebecca, "he could lose parts of his face?"

Yes, all the dark blotches could, in time, turn necrotic.

Dr. Kleinman had previous patients who had lost patches from the nose, cheeks, and ears. The photographs would offer a baseline for potential plastic surgery. At the moment, Dr. Kleinman did not mention that the greatest tissue loss would likely involve Andrew's limbs.

When it didn't get in the nurses' way, Rebecca kept her hand on Andrew. "Mommy's here," she kept saying. Rebecca got to thinking about the time he was born. It was February 5, 1991, at 11:18 at night. It was so short and easy a labor they had to wake her up: "Mrs. Bateson. It's time to push." Afterward, she felt she didn't even deserve flowers. He weighed eight pounds, nine ounces, and turned out to be an easy baby. Nothing much bothered him. He didn't walk until fifteen months, but Rebecca thought he delayed it on purpose. Andrew was a speed crawler, and seemed to think walking would slow him down. Once he ruined his Easter outfit by crawling the whole day in it.

Andrew entered the "twos" at a year and a half. To keep the kids happy while she cooked, Rebecca put kitchen implements in the lower drawers for them to discover. Her daughter, Erin, would take out one spoon and one baster; Andrew had to pull out every item.

When he was four, the family visited Rebecca's father in a nursing home. Andrew put his head through a porch railing and got stuck. They needed to smear Vaseline on the balusters to get him out. As soon as he was free, he ran into the bathroom and locked the door. The custodian had to unlock it with a master key. They found Andrew inside, putting toilet paper in the bowl, flushing it and watching it unravel off the spool. He thought that was about the neatest thing he had ever seen. The nursing home people did not seem sorry to see the Batesons leave that day.

Not long after, they were in Boothbay, Maine, at the home of Rebecca's uncle, a seventy-eight-year-old retired surgeon. Andrew walked inside and locked everyone out of the house. Her uncle spent a long time trying to talk Andrew into opening the door. He finally complied, but on his own schedule. Andrew liked running the show.

At home, Scott and Rebecca had to take all the interior door locks out of the house. They glued the dead bolts open. Still, any knob Andrew could touch, he would touch. The same went for light switches. If they were on, Andrew walked around turning them off. If off, he turned them on.

Rebecca's mind went back and forth to such thoughts as she watched the doctors and nurses do their work.

Perhaps four hours had gone by since Andrew had come up from the ER. Dr. Kleinman had barely left the room. Usually doctors gave care from afar, through phones, charts, and nurses. The PICU was different. You could not hand it off. That was truer with meningococcemia than just about any other illness.

Kleinman's title was intensivist. Hasbro had three others, all women, making it the only PICU in the country with an all-female attending staff. Each spent one seven-day week per month on the floor. During that week, it was common for Kleinman to make it home only for sleep. Even then, she was routinely awakened by calls from residents, sometimes up to ten a night. That is why there was a need for weekly rotation.

Although her children were the sickest in the hospital, Kleinman thought this a more hopeful place than adult ICUs, where patients were often at the end of their lives. On the pediatric side, most kids recovered and lived normally. The mortality rate was under 10 percent. Andrew Bateson was in a different category. When a meningococcemia patient presented with spreading purpura and shock, Kleinman had found the death rate approached 80 percent.

The next shift of nurses came in. Claire Piette was among them. She saw the number of people in room 228 and did not need to ask. Meningococcemia was among few diseases where the pace of ongoing care was akin to an ER trauma admission.

The instructions from Dr. Kleinman were continuous.

"Give me a 20-cc-per-kilo bolus of normal saline," she said.

"Titrate to maintain systolic blood pressure greater than 90."

"Let's up the dobutamine to 10 mikes."

She tried to anticipate.

"Why don't we tell the blood bank to get another two units of plasma thawed?" Kleinman said. "I'm sure we're going to need them in an hour."

She asked how long it had been since Andrew's last blood gas. Several minutes.

"Let's send a calcium with the next blood draw." Meningococcemia drained calcium, and without it Andrew's heart would not work well.

Kleinman wanted more accurate central venous pressure readings. "Can you hook that transducer to a CVP monitor?"

She instructed another bolus of albumin, 150 cc's. The nurses started it.

She checked the monitors. BP was 75 over 30. "His pressure's down. Let's give another bolus of saline."

Normally, as the leader of a resuscitation effort, Kleinman delegated tasks, but in this case she often stepped in.

"You've been at that for ten minutes," she said respectfully to a resident. "We need that line in. I'm going to try it myself."

Later, a nurse said Andrew still needed BP support. "What do you want to do?" she asked.

"Let's try albumin again," Dr. Kleinman said. "This time, 200 cc's." The nurse twisted a big syringe into an interlock and pushed in the albumin.

Although in a coma, Andrew became restless. That bothered the nurses, who didn't like to see a patient unsettled.

"What do you want to do in terms of sedation?" one asked.

Dr. Kleinman ordered two drugs. "Let's run some drips of morphine and Versed," she said.

Her tone was calm. It was how Kleinman reacted to stress.

"His drips aren't holding him," said a nurse. "Which one would you like to increase?"

"Why don't we give him a bolus of morphine and boost the drip to 3 milligrams an hour."

Dr. Kleinman examined Andrew's arms and legs. "I have pulses in the feet," she said. "I think we're making progress." Still, upon pressing his skin with her thumb, capillary refill took four seconds. Much over two was a concern.

"I wish he weren't so tachycardic," she said, noting that his heart rate was jumping around 200. "It would be reassuring if it came down."

Andrew was so in need of fluids that one nurse's sole role was administering them. Each bolus of saline lasted only fifteen minutes before his pressure dropped again; that was how quickly it leaked out inside him.

Claire thought of the parents: *These poor people really don't know what they're in for.* She saw no point in telling them. She did not think it would serve a purpose to give the Batesons the whole prediction.

One of the residents approached the parents. Andrew would likely require blood transfusions, and the team had to have a signature. Andrew's blood wasn't clotting the way it should, and he needed plasma. Rebecca and Scott looked at each other. What about AIDS, hepatitis? That was what went through their minds. Scott hesitated.

Deb Powers was there with them. "Scott," she said, "you don't have a choice here." She told him blood supplies were different now. He didn't have to worry. The parents signed the papers.

Dr. Kleinman had come to Providence seventeen years before to enroll at Brown University as an undergraduate. She grew up as an only child in St. Louis. Her father was an aeronautical engineer, her mom an elementary-school teacher. She stayed at Brown through medical school, finishing in 1987. She liked pediatric rounds the most. Many adult patients, she found, were casualties of their own self-abuse, whether it be smoking, drinking, or not wearing a seat belt. Children tended to be purer victims of what-ever brought them to the hospital and, as a doctor, Kleinman thought it was a better fit.

She became an intensivist at Hasbro, the state's new children's hospital, in August of 1995, and soon found herself handling meningococcemia cases at a surprising pace. In the past, Hasbro had seen two or three cases a year. In 1996, Kleinman saw two dozen. During some month-long stretches, a week wouldn't go by without one.

"We have another kid with meninge." It became a regular com-ment between the intensivists. They wondered when it would stop.

Because it was a reportable disease, they notified the Rhode Island Department of Health every time. Officials there were watching it, but it had not crossed the threshold for a statewide epidemic—the equivalent of 10 cases per 100,000 population. The Health Department didn't want to overreact to what might be a blip on the chart. But Kleinman and her colleagues grew anxious, as each case was quite dramatic to them. The intensivists worried it might accelerate. They thought they had a secret nobody else was willing to see.

Many patients were clustered around the city of Woonsocket. The intensivists thought it was close to an official outbreak for that area. In October of 1996, when cases there increased, the Health Department decided to vaccinate locally. Around 17,000 Woonsocket children received shots. It was a major effort. The cases stopped.

A few months later, at the start of 1997, Hasbro saw another increase, many from over the Rhode Island border in the city of Fall River, Massachusetts. More than once the intensivists remarked to each other: "Here we go again." They called the Massachusetts Department of Health, which found that the numbers fell short of a local epidemic, but were worthy of watching. The Fall River cases eventually tailed off, without vaccinations. Kleinman and her colleagues felt they had gotten lucky.

Often, the four talked about what caused the clusters. Over time, Kleinman knew, disease bacteria mutated in ways that made them more successful. Perhaps there were several such strains now in the area. Kleinman thought about another bacteria, called pneumococcus, which in some regions showed resistance to penicillin in about half the cases. To her, that reflected impressive biological scheming. It was a reason to have a healthy respect for bacteria.

Because they were in a quarantine room with full precautions required, nurses could not easily walk out, or others in. Instead, when they needed supplies they wrote requests on pieces of paper and held them to the window.

"I think we have to give 100 cc's of packed cells," said Dr. Kleinman.

A nurse wrote *prbc* and held up the sign. It stood for packed red blood cells, the kind separated from serum to eliminate unnecessary volume. Scribbling *FFP* meant they needed fresh frozen plasma. *Cryo* stood for cryoprecipitate, frozen plasma with clotting factors for patients prone to hemorrhage. *Epi* was for epinephrine. *Platelets* was just that; they used no abbreviation for it.

They kept other supplies inside so they would have them at hand: saline, albumin, and big two-ounce syringes to push fluids or medications into the lines. Those went in much faster than a drip.

Kleinman often summed up Andrew's status to keep everyone focused. "He's oxygenating well," she said, "though he's got some metabolic acidosis, so perfusion isn't optimal." The team waited for her decision on what to do about it.

"I'd like to see his acidosis improve," she said. "We should probably manipulate his drips some, see if we can get better perfusion." She gave instructions for that.

Increasingly, Kleinman worried about Andrew's extremities. His body, beset by toxins, continued to generate millions of tiny clots, which soon filled the endpoint arteries in his feet and hands. Kleinman noticed a visible line at each mid-calf below which the skin was blue. The blood there had sludged, congealing like putty.

At the same time, Andrew was entering a state called DIC, disseminated intravascular coagulation. Having first overclotted, he was now running out of platelets for necessary clotting. That caused him to start bleeding out into his tissues. One of the most noticeable places this happened was beneath the skin, which was why the purpura continued to spread.

His fever persisted, his renal function continued downhill, and his heart rate often soared to 200.

Kleinman thought about how this disease seemed to find every conceivable way to ruin the body. It left her with a lot to manage.

Rebecca became aware that the staff was careful with what they said around her. She began to watch the eyes of the doctors and nurses for clues to their thinking. She studied the way they looked at the monitors, and at each other. That told Rebecca whenever something wasn't right.

Dr. Kleinman stepped out of the room a moment, sat at the nurses' station, and dialed home. Gary answered. He worked as a paramedic in Providence, and was about to become emergency coordinator with the U.S. Public Health Service in Boston.

"Things are still pretty unstable here," she told him. "I'm not sure if I'm going to be able to leave at all."

"Are you okay?"

He was referring to her morning sickness. They had found out about the pregnancy only the week before.

She told him she was fine, which was not altogether accurate. Both knew she worked seven-day shifts and had six to go on this one.

"Try to take it easy," he said. "Try to take care of yourself. Get something to eat."

"They have Saltines in the ICU," she told him. There was a jar of them there for kids. From time to time, Dr. Kleinman snitched a few for herself. As she told Gary good-bye, she thought briefly about what she might have done had this been a normal holiday. With luck, she would have been home by early afternoon. Maybe she and Gary would have worked around the yard, or gone shopping.

Later, Kleinman would phone the other three intensivists. She reached Dr. Mindy Morin first. "We have another meninge," Kleinman said of Andrew. "He's real sick." She described the still-spreading purpura. Afterward, Morin talked about it with the other two intensivists, Dr. Linda Snelling and Dr. Pam Feuer. Given Kleinman's description, they believed his survival was unlikely. But at least he was among doctors with experience in this, thought Dr. Snelling. Advanced meningococcemia was not the kind of disease you wanted to find your way on. There wasn't time for that.

Andrew's blood pressure would not hold up. They continued to pour fluid into him, pushing vasopressors to get his vessels to hold on to it. Nurse Claire Piette thought about how much more extreme this was than treating routine shock from dehydration. With that, you seldom had to go to dopamine. Even if it was blood loss from a car accident, you usually just hung a bag of saline or plasma and kids stabilized. With most young children, five cc's per kilo would do it. If they were really shocky, maybe you hit them with 400 cc's, about a half liter. That was a big bolus. Andrew was at four times that and counting. He had gotten two-plus liters, the equivalent of his entire blood supply. He now had double the circulatory fluid for a child of forty-five pounds. Much of this volume had bled out of his vessels, pressing against his organs. Kleinman worried that with so heavy a chest it would become a problem for the vent to blow air into Andrew's lungs. Nor could they just dial the vent higher, as that would damage his air sacs.

If he became much more bloated, fluid could begin breaching his lungs, the start of pulmonary edema. That could lead to Kleinman's greatest concern, acute respiratory distress syndrome. Usually, ARDS caused the lungs to fail. They filled with fluid, blocking air absorption. Just about everything that could go wrong with lungs did. When a child with meningococcemia developed ARDS, it was often the end. Lungs became so waterlogged that, ultimately, fluid poured back out of the very ventilator tube you were trying to push air into. Oxygen levels then crashed, and the child became hypoxic. Kleinman had watched children progress to that stage with less severe forms of the disease than Andrew had. "If you have a family priest," Dr. Kleinman told the Batesons, "you might want to have him come."

Chapter 3

"We're still not out of the woods . . ."

The Reverend Joe Escobar didn't want to alarm Scott and Rebecca, but he felt he should ask. "I think it would be good if
we prayed." They were standing by Andrew's bed. It was
nighttime.

"That's not last rites," Rebecca said, "is it?"

Father Joe had spent seven years as assistant pastor at St. Pius,
the Batesons' church in Providence. He had been transferred to a
different parish a year ago. He was thirty-seven. He had spent this
July Fourth at the beach with relatives. Late that afternoon, he
phoned his new rectory for messages. There were two from former
parishioners, both about Andrew. The messages told Father Joe to
call Hasbro Children's.

Yes, a nurse said, Andrew was critical.

Father Joe was dressed in shorts and a T-shirt and did not have
his clerics with him. He had never ministered to the ill this way. He
asked the nurse if he had time to stop home; she advised he come
straight to the hospital.

Scott Bateson saw Father Joe through the window of Andrew's
room and came out. He began to speak, but was overcome. Father
Joe grew up in the same East Providence neighborhood Scott was
from. He used to wait on Scott's parents when he clerked at a con-

venience store there. Father Joe put his arms around Scott. The two stood silently like that for a few seconds.

Father Joe asked how Andrew was.

"I just don't know," Scott said. "They're hitting us with a lot of stuff."

Father Joe gowned up and walked inside. He had no experience with bacterial meningitis. Although Father Joe knew Andrew well, the bruising and bloating made him unrecognizable. He was one of the young kids at St. Pius Church, always running around. He never sat still, especially during Mass.

Father Joe understood hospitals, having spent time as a chaplain at Sloan-Kettering in New York. He saw that Andrew was ventilated. Briefly, he read the monitors, but thought you can discern more by looking at faces. He studied the nurses' eyes and picked up on silences. He had a sense there was a question of living or dying.

"You can say a prayer," Rebecca told Father Joe, "but you're not going to give him his last rites."

Father Joe explained it was seldom called that anymore. The church regarded it as a healing ritual.

Fine, Rebecca said, as long as God understood they weren't giving up.

There were three nurses in the room. They paused to join the circle. Father Joe placed a hand on Andrew's arm to include him. He asked the Lord to be with them. He asked wisdom for the intensive-care staff. Father Joe felt there wasn't time for an Our Father or Hail Mary. He made the sign of the cross. Rebecca noticed that even as they prayed, the nurses watched Andrew's monitors.

Rev. Ken Letoile was the pastor at St. Pius. Father Joe called to let him know about Andrew. Hospital work was a stretch for Father Ken. Some priests could walk into a solemn gathering and lighten the mood, but that wasn't him. Father Ken knew that no one would accuse him of being the life of the party. It was especially hard for him to connect with parishioners he didn't know well, like the

Batesons. Although he had baptized Andrew, he ministered to 1,600 families.

He retrieved the small black case that contained the three essential things: prayers for the sick, a vessel of anointing oil, and a pyx for the Eucharist. He felt nervous as he drove over in his '91 Honda Civic. He hoped God would help him find the right words.

Father Ken was fifty years old. His dad had owned a Rhode Island auto-body shop; his mother was its bookkeeper. He had four younger sisters. He had gone to Catholic schools in Providence, then nearby Providence College, and now, after several out-of-state assignments, was back as a priest in the same church where he had been an altar boy.

"Let's join hands," Father Ken said. They surrounded the bed. Rebecca touched Andrew's shoulder. A yellow gown covered Father Ken's clerics. He spoke through a hospital mask. "Deliver Andrew, Lord, from every evil. Grant him peace this day, free him and protect him, for we wait in joyful hope for the coming of You, Our Savior, Jesus Christ."

The room blipped with the sounds of machines. The parents responded: "For the kingdom, the power, the glory are Yours."

Father Ken unzipped his black leather case and reached for the pyx, a flat metal container the shape of a pocket watch. He took off the lid. "Rebecca, the body of Christ." She crossed one hand over the other. He placed the Eucharist in her palm. The ventilator hissed.

"Scott, body of Christ."

The nurses worked around them. Andrew was unable to receive, having not yet made his first communion, so Father Ken connected him to the Eucharist by touching his forehead. He had to be careful because of the dark lesions. In illness, Father Ken believed, the need to be with the body of Christ was acute. In his view, it conveyed a power even greater than prayer or the reading of the Bible.

Monitors continued to beep. Father Ken thought it important to pray silently for caregivers, as Christ worked through them:

"Jesus, send Your healing love to Andrew. Free him from this illness and guide the doctors and nurses."

He concluded out loud. "Jesus, be with us in this hospital room. Continue to watch over Andrew. Bring peace to his family and send Your healing love."

"Amen."

He told Scott and Rebecca he would stop by tomorrow. The parents were grateful for the priests' visits. At this point, they thought prayer was as important as medicine.

Father Ken drove back to St. Pius in the dark. More than in most hospital visits, he had felt an intense presence of Christ at Andrew's bedside. He walked upstairs to his priory bedroom, carrying the black leather case with him. Though he lived above the "store," he liked to keep the case at hand in the event of a late call.

As he got ready for sleep, he went over his day, thanking God for the graces He provided, and His forgiveness, as Father Ken would put it, for anything he had blown. His thoughts remained on Andrew. He had a strong sense that Christ wanted to work through him on behalf of this child. It was so vivid it kept him awake for a bit. It was a profound moment of feeling called.

It occurred to Monica Kleinman that she was less aware of her morning sickness. Everyday concerns, such as eating and sleeping, faded in a crisis.

Treating a child in the acute phase of meningococcemia was the greatest critical-care task in her experience. There was no magic medicine to give. But this was what she had been trained for, a stressful resuscitation involving skill and judgment. Kleinman saw herself as doing battle with the disease. Here was an adversary that affected every organ in the body. The challenge was being a good enough doctor to stay ahead of it.

She asked the nurses to start a drip of epinephrine, stronger than dopamine, to give some extra help to Andrew's heart.

· · ·

The latest bloods arrived. They showed Kleinman that Andrew's body had used up all his clotting factors. He was now in danger of spontaneous bleeding, externally from his IV sites, or internally from anywhere, perhaps even his brain. With his circulatory fluids already leaking out inside, this would be a further disaster. One choice was to give him platelets, more coags, but that could further clot off his arms and legs.

Dr. Kleinman's choices were difficult. Her patient needed contradictory therapies: clotting factors on the one hand, and drugs to counteract clotting on the other. Kleinman talked with her colleague Mindy Morin about it. Would more platelets dampen the fire? Or feed it? The two went back and forth.

This, Kleinman thought, was the dilemma of meningococcemia. There was seldom a clear choice. That was innate to medicine in general; most treatments carried risk. Aspirin could harm the stomach, Tylenol the liver. But usually the choices weren't as dramatic as this. Should she save Andrew's legs or his life? Was there a way to do both? Or either?

Kleinman soon made the decision to give Andrew more platelets. He was already so starved of oxygen as to be near multi-organ failure. He couldn't afford an added bleeding problem. Kleinman asked the nurses to go ahead and hang the blood products. She hoped it wouldn't worsen the haywire clotting of his extremities. In some cases, she had even found that adding plasma calmed the body's inflammatory reaction. Perhaps they'd get lucky.

They put a bag on an IV pole and started the drip. Rebecca watched the blood go into Andrew's body. It took an hour. As soon as that one ran out, they hung a second.

Later, Rebecca noticed that they hung three blood products at one time: red cells, platelets, and plasma. They said his white count was 90,000. She asked what was normal. Around 5,000 to 10,000, they told her.

If the problem was toxins in his blood, Rebecca asked, couldn't they just give him a full transfusion? Replace his blood supply with a clean one?

The damage, Kleinman explained, had gone beyond his circulation. The blood, which was poisoned, had tainted everything it touched. It had carried toxins into his liver, his kidneys, all his organs. The whole system had become infected. You could compare it to a reservoir becoming contaminated.

Family members began to come, and then neighbors. Cindy and Mike Day lived across the street on College Road. They and the Batesons had spent the previous afternoon relaxing at a pond in the Rhode Island countryside. Andrew had been fine, running in and out of the water. At the PICU, Cindy Day wondered how any disease could move that fast. She and Mike stayed until midnight.

More people came. Joe Mullen was a neighbor and painting contractor. "My God, Scott," he said, "that's Andrew?" Scott tried to explain how the disease progressed. It left Mullen with the image of Andrew's blood having caught fire and boiled. Mullen had never seen anybody so at death's door, but, as he put it, he felt Andrew's spirit was a heck of a lot bigger than the rest of everyone else's and he would beat this with that alone. It's how Andrew had been on the block: He never slowed down once.

The waiting room was full when Maria Amaral got to Hasbro in the late afternoon. She had been friends with Rebecca since West Warwick Junior High. The two families were due to leave together the next day for a week's vacation in Waterville Valley, New Hampshire. Had Maria not been told this was Andrew's hospital room, she would not have known who it was. He appeared as if badly burned in a fire.

Jimmy Bateson, one of Scott's brothers, stared at Andrew through the window. Except for the color of Andrew's hair, Jimmy could not tell this was his nephew. "How could he live looking like this?"

he said. Deb Powers, Rebecca's eldest sister, was standing by him. "He will live," she said, then told Jimmy that while here, he had to be positive. It became a rule enforced by both sides of the family; if you weren't optimistic, you weren't welcome.

Rebecca's three sisters stood by the nurses' station. Being the eldest, Deb Powers organized assignments. Who would take the first shift? The second? The third? They worked it out that Janice would relieve Deb, who would relieve Jennifer, who would relieve Janice. It was as if each were scheduling a watch. Scott's family planned regular times too. They felt someone always needed to be there. Deb believed the power of everyone's presence would somehow help Andrew. A lot of them believed it.

Mid-evening, about eight hours after Andrew's arrival, he clamped down. For hours, his vessels had been leaking. Now, in a rebound reaction, his circulatory system went into a spasm. It further cut off Andrew's extremities. They became colder to the touch, his pulses weaker. Kleinman pressed on his leg. His capillary-refill rate took a worrisome five seconds.

"Feel his feet," Dr. Kleinman told the residents. "They're ice cold. He's clamped down."

Dr. Kleinman had no clear choices. She could back off on dopamine, hoping to loosen his vessels for the sake of his legs and hands. But if they loosened too much, it could bottom out his blood pressure.

Dr. Kleinman tried a middle ground. She continued his dopamine, at the same time starting intravenous nitroglycerin to try relaxing Andrew's spasmed vessels. She did this carefully, watching the monitor. They dialed the nitro to the maximum, but had to back off it when it threatened to push down Andrew's pressure. It didn't work well. Kleinman wasn't surprised; Andrew's body was in such a powerful vasospasm it was hard to break.

Next, she tried to dilate the vessels with amrinone. That helped only a little bit.

Kleinman settled into a pattern of constant, complex adjustments. It went like that for hours. They were at a point where medicine was as much art as science. She was not a cook, but viewed this part of her job in similar language. A pinch of this, a dash of that, a bolus of this.

Dr. Kleinman again sat down with Rebecca and Scott in the small consultation room. Andrew's condition, she said, was still critical, and would remain so. But she was impressed with the strength of his lungs. So far, they had resisted dangerous decline. That was a surprise. She'd expected Andrew to have had more problems with his ventilator. Other organs were not doing as well. She was worried about Andrew's kidneys. His body had shut off blood flow there to reserve circulation for the heart and brain. She believed his kidneys would soon fail. If so, they would have to put Andrew on dialysis. Her other big concern was his extremities. Andrew's toes were blue and his fingertips grayish. The pulses in his limbs were weak. Often, Kleinman said, meningococcemia caused some kind of extremity loss.

She did not think this registered with the Batesons.

By ten that night, the room was so full of IV poles Rebecca could barely take a step. There were always two nurses and a doctor in the room, everyone dressed in yellow isolation gowns, hats, and gloves. Dr. Kleinman seldom left. She remained calm, never yelling orders, but neither did she stop giving them.

Rebecca watched Andrew's heart rate go from 90 to 213. That happened often. The ups and downs wore on her. Every time she thought there was a turn for the better, five things turned for the worse. His blood was clotting too much, then not enough. His temperature rose, then fell. If they got a break with his pressure, his heart started to race. The room was never quiet. Despite the hour, lights remained on throughout the ICU, making it easy to forget it was night.

. . .

A new shift of nurses came in. Rebecca's sister Deb realized there was no way they could know what Andrew really looked like. He was intubated and full of lines. His arms and legs were both wrapped. He was blackened by welts and bloated. About the only recognizable part of him was a shock of hair.

Deb went to the Batesons' house, in part for clothes and toothbrushes, but also for photographs. Back at the hospital she and Rebecca put them up, taping one above Andrew's bed on the power column that ran the pumps.

"This is Andrew," announced Deb to those in the room. "This is what Andrew really looks like."

"What a handsome boy," said one of the nurses.

Every now and then the staff would glance up at the pictures.

Deb wished the family could convey more about who Andrew was. Perpetual motion, she thought, the kind of boy who is always throwing or kicking some ball. He liked to push limits. The last thing you wanted to tell him was "I don't think that's a good idea." When he was learning to ride a bike at age four, Rebecca put a stick down on the sidewalk and said he could go no farther from the house. He immediately went past it. When Rebecca asked what he was doing, Andrew said, "Oh, I thought you meant *that* stick." He saw a line as something to cross.

Once, while on Rollerblades outside Deb's house, he held on to a rope tied to his cousin's bike, and off they went. Andrew was five at the time. That same year he said he wanted his ear pierced. He got the idea from Deb's son-in-law, who wore an earring. Aunt Janice's oldest two had tattoos—one a shamrock, the other a fighting Irish leprechaun. She wished they hadn't gotten them. Andrew wished he could.

Whenever Andrew's fever spiked beyond 102, the Batesons heard a small debate. Give him Motrin? Or would that thin blood that was already leaking internally? When it got to 104, Rebecca could feel tension in the room. She asked if she could help with fans and damp cloths. The nurses got them for her. She covered her son with cool towels, occasionally wiping his face. She trained a fan on him, and from time to time changed the towels. At 2 A.M. or so, the fever began to break. There was no question in Dr. Kleinman's mind that Rebecca made the difference. We did everything we could, Kleinman thought, and then fell back on what parents have always done for fevers, and it was more effective than the expertise of the intensive care unit.

As his fever reduced, Andrew's inflammatory reaction calmed slightly. He still required fluids, but for the first time in fourteen hours Dr. Kleinman was able to pause. It made her aware of how drained she felt. She thought she should grab the chance. There would still be a senior resident at Andrew's bedside. Kleinman found an empty room and asked the nurses to wake her in two hours, earlier if anything came up. She did not have to be specific. ICU nurses were good at knowing when to worry. At 2 A.M., she lay down on a hospital bed and was quickly asleep.

Rebecca began to rub Andrew's feet. She hoped this would improve the circulation. The resident told her he wasn't sure it would help, but her son's feet were cold and Rebecca wanted to warm them. She rubbed them past 3 A.M., then four. As she did, she began to bargain. *Just let him live,* she prayed. *If You give me that, I'll deal with whatever else I have to.*

Then she thought about a time the previous October when she was going through Andrew's school backpack. He was five years old. She found a note and opened it up. It was from a neighbor girl his same age. It told him to meet in her backyard at four o'clock. Rebecca decided to intercept it. She was not interested in her son sneaking off to a romantic rendezvous at age five. That was what popped into her head as she sat sleepless in the intensive care unit.

Dr. Kleinman was awakened at four by a knock on the door. The nurse did not say anything, just gave the signal. Kleinman walked to the sink and put enough cold water on her face to help her focus.

She still had yesterday's scrubs on. Later, she hoped to take a shower and put on a new set.

Andrew looked worse to her, but his heart rate had notched down and his pressure up. She put her fingers on the radial artery of his wrist; the pulse was fuller. She wanted to believe he had turned a corner but had too much experience with this disease to trust it.

Not long after, Andrew was in full kidney failure.

His renal function had begun to deteriorate before midnight. He was retaining toxins the body was supposed to eliminate, and his urinary output had stopped. This posed a crisis because Andrew by now had gotten ten pounds of fluids, almost triple his normal blood quantity. Without kidney function, he had no way to get rid of it.

His body was so swollen even Scott and Rebecca found him hard to recognize. He did not look like their son anymore.

The monitor showed he wasn't getting enough oxygen, which meant fluid had leaked into his chest cavity and begun to compress his lungs. Dr. Kleinman felt they were heading toward ARDS. It was the right time, twelve to twenty-four hours into septic shock. She had the respiratory therapist dial up the ventilator, but if much more fluid built up it would start leaking into Andrew's air sacs. Dialysis remained the one way to filter out extra fluid. Kleinman had placed meningococcemia patients on dialysis before, but never this early.

Dr. Mindy Morin came to the PICU to check on the new meninge patient. If Andrew survived, she would be getting him the following week. The feeling in the room was tense. Dr. Morin did not like the look of his legs. The skin had a blue cast to mid-calf, as if Andrew were wearing high socks. The amount of purpura was impressive. She was not hopeful about his chances.

She and Dr. Kleinman stepped out of the room. The two were careful to hold certain talks away from the parents.

"His kidneys have shut down," Monica told Mindy. "I think

we have to start dialyzing him." There were downsides. Rerouting volume outside his body could further collapse blood pressure. And Kleinman would rather not have to insert large catheters into a child with bleeding problems. There was a risk it might further reduce blood flow to his legs, which Andrew could ill afford. On the other hand, if they did not take fluid off him he would not survive. Kleinman hoped Andrew was strong enough to take the insults dialysis was about to impose.

Kleinman prepared the parents. "The kidneys are the first thing to go," she explained, "and the last thing to come back."

The parents asked what dialysis meant for Andrew. Kleinman went over the risks. "It's just another thing we'll have to deal with," she said.

With dialysis about to be added to the mix, Dr. Kleinman decided Andrew should have a larger space. There would be more equipment now, and another nurse. Room 225 was open, so that was where he went. It took almost an hour to pack him up, another to settle him in. That was how many lines, bags, pumps, and poles there were.

Dr. Kleinman gathered a team to place Andrew on dialysis. It would involve putting two quarter-inch tubes into his upper inner thighs, huge lines for a little boy. The day before, he'd had a central line inserted in the femoral vein there as an infusion port for medications. They would need to take over that spot for the dialysis. First Kleinman moved the infusion port to his jugular. That left a now-open puncture as an entry point. Kleinman asked a resident to do the procedure on that side. The new dialysis catheter was double the size of the hole, so the resident had to make it wider. He inserted a dilator into Andrew's skin, burrowing a broader hole to his vein. He had to use force to create a path, tunneling through skin and muscle.

Kleinman now had to insert a catheter on the other upper inner thigh for the exit tube. This was a more difficult procedure since there was no existing hole. His purpura and swollen tissues made it hard to probe for a good spot. This side was riskier than a vein, arterial pressure being higher. A mistake would cause far more bleeding, especially in a child who had run out of clotting factors.

She found a pulse and, with one hand palpating it, inserted a syringe needle, pulling back the plunger until it drew a flash of blood an inch and a half in. She stopped, removed the syringe, and using a dilator, burrowed a wider passage to the artery. A jet of blood came out. In other patients Kleinman had seen the jet go across a room. Arterial pressure was that strong. They immediately clamped it off.

The process was more invasive than Rebecca expected. There was enough blood loss to require another transfusion. It was almost noon on the second day.

The nursing staff took over, connecting the lines to the dialysis machine so Andrew's blood would be routed through it in a horseshoe circuit. They looked at Kleinman and asked if she was ready.

"Go ahead."

They removed the clamps from the tubes. His blood flowed out toward the filter. Soon, a few cc's at a time, excess fluid started to drain off into a bag. This caused Andrew's blood pressure to drop, a bad turn. Kleinman chose not to intervene. She waited several more minutes. The pressure did not drop any more. Andrew had tolerated it. The filtration steadied at a rate that would draw out a half liter in twenty-four hours. That was only a fraction of what he owed them, but it was all he could support.

It appeared to Rebecca that machines, tubes, and drugs were now doing almost everything for Andrew. His lungs were taken over by a ventilator, his kidneys by dialysis. Medications were assisting his heart and circulation. He was constantly getting blood and other fluids. He was being fed through an IV. He was on a heated air mattress to control his temperature. He was receiving almost every type of critical-care support available. From time to time, they added another line or a new monitoring gauge, continuing to connect him to things.

Dr. Kleinman walked over to the nurses' station and unwrapped a pack of Saltines. She was feeling morning sickness again. Being deprived of sleep didn't help. The anesthesiologist, Rick Browning, noticed and walked up to her.

"You're not pregnant, are you?"

Kleinman smiled and calmly denied it. She wasn't public at that point. It was early in the pregnancy, and she knew a certain number are lost before the third month. She went to get herself a cup of tea.

Kleinman was increasingly worried about Andrew's feet and hands. The amount of leg discoloration was exceptional for twenty-four hours, even for the sickest meningococcemia patients. The swelling was like a tourniquet. Andrew's legs were so distended as to have hardened. It was more like touching Styrofoam than skin.

She discussed it with the other intensivists. One idea was to try fasciotomies: deep incisions in the intermuscular spaces of the leg to let the tissues expand. Kleinman decided that would cause too much bleeding. Besides, the damage was from clotting within the vessels. Fasciotomies wouldn't easily address that.

Kleinman did decide to try nitroglycerin paste, a topical stimulant that dilated blood vessels. Scott stood outside the window and watched. After a few minutes Dr. Kleinman pointed to Andrew's foot and gave a thumbs-up. Apparently there had been some reaction. Scott had a sense of hope come over him. Maybe this was an answer. The effect, however, did not last long. Back in the room, Scott touched Andrew's feet. They remained cool. That was how the hours went for him: You got your hopes up, and then . . . nothing.

There was one dramatic treatment in the literature to address such extremity blockage. It was a drug called tPA, and it was often given to heart-attack victims to dissolve clots in coronary vessels. The downside was that it could cause spontaneous bleeding in someone with platelet problems. The bleeding could take place in the GI tract or even the brain.

Dr. Kleinman thought tPA had the best chance of offering relief to Andrew's extremities. Nevertheless, she knew it could trigger bleeding severe enough to cause the patient's death. As much as she wanted to give the Batesons more hope for Andrew's limbs, Kleinman decided she shouldn't take such a gamble. This was the sort of choice she had to make.

Scott paid close attention whenever they checked Andrew's feet. He touched and tested them, trying to believe they were not getting colder. He could see that the toes on both feet had darkened but told himself, "No, it's going to come back." He believed that the mental act of sending out hope could make a difference. The pulses in Andrew's feet and legs came and went. Mostly they got weaker. It reminded Scott of a pipe that kept closing and closing.

Yet again, they sat in the consultation room. Dr. Kleinman began with the positives. Andrew's acidosis had resolved, and his blood pressure, though low, was stable. That said, here were her concerns:

"We're still not out of the woods as far as his lungs go."

She moved on. Despite all they were doing, the impaired circulation to the hands and feet was worsening.

"I don't know," she said. "I'm hoping his hands will improve."

Scott's focus was on Andrew's feet. He asked if there was hope there.

Kleinman said that blood flow had been largely blocked.

No one said anything for a moment.

"I'm sorry to keep giving you difficult news," Dr. Kleinman said, "but I've promised to be honest with you about everything."

She told them about tPA. "The danger," she said, "is it also causes bleeding." Andrew would have little tolerance for that. She was afraid tPA could kill him. There was no question in her mind that it probably would.

Rebecca seemed to be listening more than Scott. He seemed lost.

She asked if there was anything else they could try.

Yes, there was one other option. An epidural: a nerve block in the spine to relax the vessels below.

Rebecca asked how they would go about it.

They would insert a needle between the bones of the lumbar spine and push a local anesthetic. It would relax the nerves below, causing blood vessels to open slightly. There were no guarantees, given how Andrew's limbs were filled with clots. Nor could Kleinman promise it was safe; this was a needle inside the spine. But it was all she had for them. Rebecca was feeling overwhelmed by decisions. Dialysis, transfusions, epidurals—there always seemed to be another crisis, another procedure.

Dr. Kleinman picked up a sense of guilt from Scott and Rebecca. They often asked what more they could have done. In a disease where speed is important, she told them, Andrew had come in very early.

Then why was he so ill?

With meningococcemia, Kleinman said, you can't always stop the cascade once it starts. You just hope you can sustain the patient through it. Still, every minute made a difference. If the Batesons had come in an hour later, Kleinman told them, even a half hour, they might not have had anything to work with.

Kleinman talked with Dr. Mindy Morin about the epidural.

"How's his platelet count?" Morin asked.

Still low. They were transfusing him right then to boost it.

"I wouldn't touch him without a count of 50,000 or more," said Morin.

A normal count was over 150,000. Andrew's was in the low thousands, virtually nothing. At that level, the epidural could cause bleeding near the spinal cord. Neither doctor liked the procedure at this point. Still, they thought they should get ready.

Even if successful, Kleinman doubted it would save everything, but it could mean toes instead of a foot. If things got worse, maybe it could save his knees. There was no way of telling.

By midday, the infusions had built Andrew's platelet count to 50,000—a third where it should have been, but enough. Kleinman called the anesthesiologist. "Now's the time," she said. As an extra guard against bleeding, she had a nurse run a bag of platelets into Andrew while the epidural was being performed. Soon after, the color of his legs improved. The improvement reached down to his ankles and feet. You could feel the optimism in the room.

An hour or so later, the color went back to where it had been before.

By now Andrew's hands had blown up like balloons with fingertips sticking out. The nailbeds were almost black. Kleinman talked with her colleagues about an arm nerve block to relax the vessels below. To do so, they would have to insert a tube beneath each biceps, but that was crowded space, and if you hit the axillary artery it could cut off circulation; you'd lose the whole arm. Kleinman decided it was too risky.

The thought that Andrew, were he to survive, could lose hands as well as feet was really a distressing one.

From time to time, Kleinman made a point of looking at Andrew's photographs. It focused her. She thought: *That's the little boy these parents know. That's who we're working to restore.*

It helped Dr. Kleinman to have had a chance to interact with Andrew. Intensivists took a lot from even brief interchanges with patients. Most six-year-olds acted out when sick, which was understandable. Andrew had tried to be cooperative. He had been quite brave.

She remembered how, just before being sedated, Andrew asked

if he could go home. Kleinman thought how nice it would be if she could help make that happen.

Rebecca picked up all she could about Dr. Kleinman. The nurses said she'd had a hand in treating every meningitis case that had come through. Rebecca respected the way Kleinman told her the truth: calmly, but without false optimism. Clearly, Kleinman wouldn't say something was all right if it wasn't.

The consultation room was where the doctors gave the parents the latest news. It was very small and decorated in mauve. In Scott's mind, not a lot that was good happened in there. The next time they met there with Kleinman, her focus was Andrew's extremities.

In most cases as advanced as this, Kleinman said, she had seen tissue loss. It could be toes, a fingertip, or maybe much more.

Scott found such statements hard to grasp. With all the hospital's talent and technology they couldn't improve this?

Kleinman explained that Andrew's vessels had been blocked and perhaps ruined. Once that happened, it was hard to reestablish circulation. She said there was a good chance of amputations of some kind. That was the first time she had been so resolute.

In Dr. Kleinman's eyes, Scott reacted to that word as if in clinical shock.

He asked how much.

She had seen children lose as little as toes, and as much as well above the knee. This was a possibility with Andrew.

How about his hands?

It could be fingertips, but some children lost arms to the shoulder. It was a possible result of meningococcemia.

Scott fell silent. It became hard to engage him in conversation. He was not hostile, but thoroughly withdrawn. His reaction was even worse than the first day, when Kleinman questioned whether Andrew would live. She had seen similar responses in the past. The idea of a child growing up with amputations can be a paralyzing image to a parent.

Rebecca continued to rub Andrew's feet, trying to warm them. She thought back to the time he had tried to call her bluff. Andrew had always been headstrong. Whenever they got in an argument he would say, "I'm going to get a new mom."

All right, she finally told him, get in the car. They would go to the playground, and he would have a good selection.

"Fine," he answered. "Let's go." That was Andrew. If you tried to one-up him, he would one-up you better. Now Rebecca was sad about having done that. It was lousy to have told him to find another mother.

Rebecca thought back to the block. Andrew was among the youngest, but he was never shy about suggesting what game they should play. Everyone got a kick out of this little tyke telling the big kids what was on the agenda. Although Andrew learned to walk late, he did everything else early. He began Rollerblading at age three. Sometimes they took him to an indoor rink that had laser tag upstairs. The way he explained it to people, there was like a suit thing, and you got a gun and had to shoot everybody. And then you had a battle, and the person who got shot the most was out. Also, you got your power back from this big thing, but you had to press a little thing on it first. That was laser tag. Andrew could play for hours.

Rebecca counted the intravenous pumps. There were twenty-eight, piggybacked two and three high. She looked at the nasogastric tube, the hookups for kidney filtration, and all the monitors. This was some rigmarole, Rebecca thought.

Sometimes, Rebecca pictured Andrew sitting on the Harley bicycle he had gotten the previous Christmas. Although it was too big, every week or so he would try to ride it again. Rebecca told the nurses that once the machines were taken out of the room she would bring in that bike. She wanted Andrew to wake up and see it. She assumed that might not be possible, but it was nice to think about.

Often Rebecca focused on the dialysis setup. Slowly, it filtered the excess fluid Andrew had aboard. It did so slowly, a drop at a time. Any quicker would stress Andrew's system. For long minutes, Rebecca just watched the drops.

She also watched the Pulseox device that measured blood oxygen saturation. That told whether the respirator was doing its job. It was supposed to read close to 100 percent, but sometimes it dipped into the 80s. She stared at the monitor as if mesmerized. It reminded her of watching CNN during a war.

Despite all the visitors, Rebecca felt alone. Perhaps it was because of Scott. At first he had kept an arm around her, but now he had pulled away.

She found herself missing her parents in a manner she had not felt before. Rebecca's mother had died soon after Erin was born, and her father a year before Andrew got sick. She was thinking about them more now than she had in years.

She wished they were there to hold her. She had thought that was going to be her husband. But maybe she was being unfair to Scott. It had not yet been two days.

At this stage in the disease, there was no book for Dr. Kleinman to go to. She looked to the other intensivists as advisers. All had been through this. Dr. Pam Feuer considered meningococcemia the worst of infections. She recalled earlier cases, like the child who had cardiac arrest three times the first day. One little girl was sitting up upon arrival, but developed purpura and ran out of platelets. She began bleeding from many sites. Her lungs filled with fluid until they were unable to ventilate her, despite dialing the machine to its maximum. She had come in mid-morning and died by 5 P.M. They had all seen children with meningococcemia code. They were able to bring them back, but only temporarily. Every one that had arrested eventually went on to die.

They talked about the differences between Andrew and the girl who had come in the day before him. Why was his case so much more severe? Perhaps Andrew had a more aggressive strain. Then again, there was no way to predict which way a case would turn. They didn't have all the answers.

As she weighed what to do, Dr. Kleinman thought about the nature of this bacteria. Under a microscope meningococcus appeared as two circles stuck together. It was a more opportunistic bacteria than most, even reckless in how it took advantage of the body. Unlike other parasites, meningococcus often killed the host it took over. There was no logic to it. It was simply voracious. Once it colonized a human, it ate and bred and multiplied, feeding off the sugar in the blood. Toxins were its waste products.

Dr. Kleinman did not view meningococcemia as scheming; it was more like a puzzle to decipher. Were she a parent of a child with the disease, she imagined she would think about it differently.

Chapter 4

"Don't you dare give up on my son . . ."

D r. Kleinman had been at the hospital thirty-six hours; she had slept for two. The second evening she decided to leave for home around 7 P.M. She told the residents to call for any reason.

She sat down to dinner with her husband, Gary. "Is this one of those times you just want me to listen," he asked, "or should I give you my thoughts?"

"I want you just to listen."

He nodded. "How's your kid doing?" He knew there had been just one keeping her there; that was all it took.

Monica said it remained tough going. Andrew came into the PICU talking, and three hours later was on a vent. His rate of decline had been impressive.

"At least he's survived so far," said Gary.

She remarked on the number of meninge cases they had gotten this year. This one, she said, was among the most challenging. "I hope the phone doesn't ring," she said, "but it probably will."

Gary nodded. "I know."

She ate as much as she could, which was little, and went to sleep soon after. Several calls did come in. None were crises, but Monica had no problem being awakened, having become involved with this little boy.

...

The next morning, the third day, she left for the hospital at six-thirty, stopping for doughnuts on the way. As she drove, Kleinman thought about her decision on tPA, the clot-breaking drug. She wished they could have used it, but she didn't second-guess that. The risk of bleeding out was just too high. As she pulled into the parking lot, she hoped Andrew's legs would look better. Perhaps the epidural had helped. That was emotion speaking, though. Kleinman was not optimistic.

In the room, she examined Andrew's legs. They were cold, his toes almost black. The color demarcation at mid-calf was clearer than before. His feet looked like those of severe frostbite victims. His hands had worsened too. Although he was in an induced coma, she spoke to him. "Good morning, Andrew. It's Dr. Kleinman. I'm going to listen to your lungs. You're getting better. Keep fighting."

Dr. Kleinman again sat with the Batesons. Scott asked about Andrew's kidneys. His son now had no function there at all. What was going to happen? Kleinman said that with kids, kidneys that failed from shock usually recovered. But they would not know for some time. Others in the PICU had told Scott you can never tell.

Scott and Rebecca then asked if Andrew would live.

Kleinman assured them again that when she could look them in the eye and say their son would survive, she would.

Dr. Kleinman called for an orthopedic surgeon. Dr. Donna Paccica was covering for Dr. Charles D'Amato. Kleinman met her outside the room. The epidural, she explained, had provided transient improvement, but the lower limbs were still dying from lack of oxygen.

"Donna," Kleinman asked, "do you have any other thoughts?"

No, it seemed to her they'd considered everything.

"Do you agree tPA is too risky?"

"Yes."

They chatted some more. There was nothing else available that had promise. It was a solemn exchange. It was hard for Kleinman to face that she had run out of ways to help. In difficult cases, when she felt an outcome was getting beyond her control, Kleinman would say a silent prayer. Usually it was brief, centered on asking God to help her help a child. There were moments now with Andrew when Kleinman offered such a prayer.

Often, there was no conversation in the room. Scott or Rebecca sat by Andrew while the nurses worked. The ventilator made constant, rhythmic sounds, and the heart monitor ticked. If the rate jumped too much, it triggered an alarm. Other alarms let the staff know when a bag of fluid or plasma was getting low. If Andrew's blood pressure changed, which was often, still another alarm signaled. All day that was the backbeat.

Rebecca worried that the machine noise would get on Andrew's nerves. She thought he should hear something more soothing. She chose a CD called *Evening Passages* from a selection brought by a relative, and put it on a portable player. It was piano music by Ed Van Fleet. It was quite tranquil. She was sure Andrew could hear it.

When Scott and Rebecca weren't at Andrew's bedside, they often retreated to the family waiting room. It had two vinyl couches, two vinyl chairs, and fluorescent fixtures overhead. There was a coffeemaker in constant use, often all night. Next to it was a bathroom with a shower. A television mounted on the far wall was usually on at low volume. The carpet was grayish green, the ceiling tiles off-white. The room was rectangular, the longest wall lined with picture windows overlooking Hasbro's circular drive. The view beyond stretched to the highway, and past that, to downtown Providence. Scott would stand there and just stare.

He eyed the low stone wall by the entrance below and remembered another time they had been there. A few years before, Rebecca's father had been in a rehabilitation center on the Rhode Island Hospital campus next door. During a visit the family had brought him outside in a wheelchair, stopping by that stone wall. Next to it, a lawn sloped to the sidewalk. Erin and Andrew began to roll down the grass. When they reached bottom, they ran back up and rolled again. They kept at it a good fifteen minutes. Finally the parents talked them into continuing the walk.

They had all gone by the front of Hasbro, looking at little works of art on display by the windows. Scott said that it was nice to have such a place close to home. "But I hope we never have to use it, guys," he added. They began to stroll back. The kids rolled down the hill again, having a ball. They didn't want to leave. Now, in the family room, Scott thought of that memory and how much he wished he could have that day back.

The rash seemed at last to have stopped spreading, though to Rebecca it didn't appear to have anywhere else to go. Andrew was covered. They told Rebecca the skin would soon start to blister as if after a burn. Bacteria entering at any of those breaks could introduce infection, which would exacerbate his septic shock. They began to culture his blood regularly, checking for new bacteria.

To Rebecca, night was the hardest. The machine noises seemed louder then, there being fewer other noises to blunt them. There were two chairs in Andrew's room. One was a vinyl rocker, the other a vinyl recliner. The chairs often served as the parents' beds. Rebecca was unable to sleep well in them. At best, she dozed.

By the third night, Rebecca thought the exhaustion would catch up to her and she would sleep hard, but she didn't. Perhaps, she thought, she was on greater alert after daytime hours. Andrew's vital signs seemed to waver more at night. His temperature rose and he was more unsettled. Rebecca focused on all the machines. She was now able to tell by sound alone whether Andrew was having a problem. Often such changes registered when she was dozing, and she would open her eyes. Outside the room, the rest of the hospital was in sleep mode. People went home and time seemed to slow. The corridors outside the PICU were quiet. That made nights harder, too. Rebecca looked forward to morning.

Sometimes, upon waking, she forgot where she was. She would try to get her bearings as if she were in their bedroom at home on College Road. The room back home was painted blue and had two cherry bureaus. On the walls there was a picture of a breakfast tray on a bed, and another of a girl in a field of flowers. From the hospital chair, she would look for those pictures, thinking she had dreamed the illness. Then she'd see the monitor and instinctively check Andrew's heart rate and pulse, his blood pressure, respiration, and temperature. She eyed the clock, waiting for dawn.

On the fourth day, Kleinman asked Mindy Morin to cover so she could keep an appointment with her obstetrician. They did an ultrasound. She and Gary saw a little nine-millimeter creature with a beating heart. Then she went back to the unit.

Rebecca heard a rumor that Dr. Kleinman was pregnant. She had suspected. When Kleinman took off her mask, she appeared drained and nauseous; Rebecca recognized the look. Kleinman had crackers in her pocket and seemed sleep-deprived, but almost never left Andrew's side. That said something to Rebecca.

That same day Rebecca saw a pea-sized bubble on Andrew's left forearm. She asked what that was.

"This is when it starts," said Dr. Kleinman.

The skin affected by purpura was starting to die. Everyone now had to be especially diligent about precautions. If you left the room, even briefly, you couldn't reenter without putting on new gowns, gloves, and masks. Rebecca went through only four sets a day; that was how infrequently she stepped out. It was the same for Scott. They were at Andrew's bedside twenty-two hours out of twenty-four, gowned throughout. It got quite warm in there. The two spent most of those hours standing so as not to get in the way of the nurses and doctors.

. . .

Rebecca missed being able to touch Andrew. Holding him was not possible, there being too many lines and hookups. Nor could she touch him with her own fingers, since latex gloves were part of required precautions. Rebecca also missed her daughter, Erin, who was staying with relatives or neighbors. The loss of both children made Rebecca feel as though she were in withdrawal. She began to doubt her parental instincts. How else was a mother to support her child if not through touch?

At the end of the fourth day, around midnight, she found herself rocking in the bedside chair. Her sister Deb was there with her. Rebecca began to cry. "I have to hold him," she said. "I have to touch him."

All Deb could say was "You'll have your time. We all miss him." It was odd to talk about missing a child who was right next to them.

Often, Rebecca asked Dr. Kleinman if Andrew would survive. Kleinman told her she was not yet able to predict.

Rebecca and Scott went to the doctors' lounge for a meeting. Rebecca noticed that lately, she and her husband were sitting at opposite ends of the couch. This time, it was yet another round of doctors saying they expected Andrew to continue downhill.

Afterward, Scott walked out the door in his own direction. He was tired of being told how bad things were going to be. Ever since Andrew got sick, every day had been "This is yours, take it." It made him angry.

He wasn't aware that it came out toward Rebecca, or that he was pulling away from her. It was not like he woke up and said "I'm not going to offer her any comfort." But what comfort? Whenever he turned around it was bad news. He considered it dishonest to put on an optimistic front. Scott wasn't the kind to whistle cheerfully at such a time.

Rebecca expected that Scott would eventually be more present to her. She thought: *He'll rescue me soon enough.*

...

Rebecca grew protective of what Andrew heard. She was convinced that at some level he was registering things. Kleinman and the nurses were always respectful of that, but not everyone was. Younger doctors came in and started reeling off their analyses and concerns.

"Excuse me," Rebecca said, "can we take this outside?"

The residents looked at her with surprise, as if to imply, "Ma'am, your child's in a coma." They did not say as much, though, and, after assessing Rebecca's resolve, retreated.

Scott noticed that Andrew's right foot was the one they were most worried about. They checked it more often for pulses. It was getting cooler. Scott asked Dr. Kleinman how she felt about it. She never pulled punches on such questions. She said there would be some loss, at least some toes. It could be much more.

They began to put a sound sensor on the ankle. It reminded Scott of one that had amplified Andrew's heartbeat when Rebecca was pregnant with him. They needed such a device now to find his pulse. During that test Scott heard nothing else, not the respirator, or people talking, or pumps pushing. He just listened for the sound of that pulse. Sometimes he could hear it fine. Then it got low, or it wouldn't be there at all. Then it came back again. Rebecca focused on it too. When there was no pulse sound she wanted to believe it was the technician.

A kidney specialist had been checking regularly on Andrew. Scott asked what they should expect.

"With these kinds of injuries," the specialist said, "you don't know. We're not sure how much his kidneys will come back." Maybe 50 percent, he said; maybe 40.

Scott asked what that would mean for Andrew. Was he going to be sick all his life? Need dialysis regularly?

No, the doctor said, but he would have to be careful about things other people don't think about, particularly diet. His kidneys would be fragile.

Scott pictured what guys like to do when they get older—have a beer, for example. Or carefree eating. You name it. Andrew, it seemed, would not be capable of handling such things.

The specialist had to leave. Scott found it hard to grasp what was happening here. What kind of disease was this? Perfectly good kidneys, and then, days later, Andrew was like an elderly person with half-ruined organs. He had so many possible deficits already, and here was one more.

A television was mounted high on the wall of Andrew's room. They seldom turned it on. Scott got to thinking about how Andrew was not the kind to veg out in front of the TV, at least if there was something happening outside, which there usually was, it being that kind of block. Right in the middle of a show Andrew would be up and gone. And he never just walked, even across their small living room; he was in too much of a hurry. Andrew, thought Scott, just wasn't a sit-still kind of kid. Well, when playing Nintendo maybe, but that was it.

By the fifth day, Andrew looked like a burn victim. He had hundreds of blisters, many of them rupturing. His body temperature dropped, and they had to turn up the room to eighty-five degrees. The threat of infection became greater. The staff and parents perspired inside their precaution garments.

The nurses began wound cleaning. Rebecca left the room, having been told it was an awful process. Scott said he wanted to stay. The nurses urged him to reconsider, but he felt Andrew would know he was there and be comforted by that.

They methodically laid out sealed implements on trays, careful to maintain a sterile field. The nurses then removed the gauze from Andrew's body and began scrubbing off the dead skin. They were not able to be gentle. If they did not remove all necrotic material, it could cause a secondary infection. Most burn victims died of opportunistic invaders like klebsiella or pseudomonas. It was what Kleinman now worried about most.

Before the scrubbing session the nurses upped Andrew's sedation, giving him more ketamine and morphine through the catheter in his neck. The nurses encouraged such strong sedation since they were convinced that even comatose kids had some awareness of pain. Once, as they began scrubbing Andrew's wounds, Scott saw his eyes open wide. That was strange to Scott. On those rare occasions when Rebecca was there for the scrubbing, she watched Andrew's face closely, but it was expressionless. She could only hope he was not feeling this.

The nurses started with each arm, then his chest, stomach, and legs. They rolled Andrew onto his side and scoured his back. They scrubbed his skin until it bled. Once done, they reexamined him from his forehead down. They did not want to miss even the tiniest infected sore. The hardest part for Scott was when they got to Andrew's face. The whole right side of it had turned black.

"Andrew," Scott said, "Dad's here." He said he would stay no matter what procedures they did to him. That was Scott's whole thing, staying near his son.

It took three nurses a full hour to finish. Afterward, they spread Silvadene on the scrubbed areas. It had the look of Noxzema. Andrew was all but covered in white. Then they covered the Silvadene with dressings. They had to do this whole procedure twice a day.

Late that fifth night, Andrew developed a fever. His white count went up, and his septic shock deepened. Dr. Kleinman was at home when a resident called, saying they assumed the cause was a skin-based infection.

"We're worried about Andrew," the resident said. They were thinking of starting dopamine again. Did Kleinman think they should broaden his antibiotics? Cover for a new infection?

She told the residents to reculture him. And meanwhile, yes, put him on vancomycin and ceftazidime—big guns for infections picked up in hospitals. Kleinman had long guessed Andrew would have problems like this. It happened to burn patients, too. He had probably picked up some bacteria, staph maybe, or pseudomonas, a particularly bad player.

How was his pressure?

Continuing to drop, even though they'd given him boluses.

All right, she said, go ahead and start dopamine.

She instructed them to call again if there were more problems. As she hung up, she thought about how you can never exhale when dealing with meningococcemia.

They did not call, but Dr. Kleinman was in early the next morning, the sixth day. As it turned out, the blood cultures did not grow out new bacteria. She worried that something could be in there somewhere, so she kept up the antibiotics. Gradually, the flare-up calmed.

The experience left Scott on edge. Whenever Andrew's heart rate or blood pressure climbed, he started asking why. Could Andrew be having another infection? All they could say was that they would know soon.

Scott stared at the monitors. He had gotten good at reading them. If the Pulseox said oxygen saturation was down, that was serious, perhaps a sign of ventilator problems. You had to respond right away, make sure the breathing tube wasn't kinked or plugged with secretions. A normal patient had a 95-to-100-percent sat rate. An asthma patient might be in the high 80s. Much lower than that got to be problematic. That's where Andrew often was.

Scott leaned close to his son. "The doctors are doing all they can for you, bud," he said. He told Andrew not to be afraid.

"You're very sick," Scott said, "but you're going to fight. You're getting better."

After several hours he left the floor for the cafeteria. That was one of three places he went, the garden and the chapel being the other two. Neither parent went home or off the grounds. If Scott was away from the room for even a half hour, he began to miss Andrew. It was strange; it wasn't as if they were able to interact. He wondered if, in an odd way, this was making a better father of him.

Seeing morning come was a good feeling to Scott. Dawn felt like you were starting fresh. Maybe the new day would bring something better. But it seemed that every few hours there were just more negatives. Scott never knew where they would come from. It could be Andrew's toes looking worse, or new kidney concerns. One specialist said this could affect his growth plates, causing life-long problems with his joints. It was one more thing in an endless row of things to worry about.

At times Scott felt like Andrew was in a box and the doctors were in another box, unable to reach him. At other times Scott felt like he was outdoors wearing clothing that could not get wet, and then it started to rain. Scott imagined himself running and dodging, but there was no dry place. It poured harder and harder, and would not stop.

People told Scott he needed to get away, at least for a few hours. They suggested he go home, relax, take a shower. He'd feel better. Scott declined. Home was a twenty-minute drive. There was no way he was going that far away.

How about a restaurant, then? One meal.

Scott begged off. It was a whole different frame of mind. It was like he was in a chunk taken out of normal life. That was where he was living, in this chunk. It was a place that had nothing to do with what came before or after. Those parts of his life were just out there somewhere, and he wasn't interested in them. The only thing clear to Scott was that he was going to stay near Andrew.

Once some friends tried hard to pin him down.

"You have to take a break," they said. "Go home. Go out."

"I'm fine," he said.

"But you should, Scott."

"I'm fine."

"It would do you good."

Scott's voice rose. "Look," he snapped, "I don't want to go out. Leave it alone." Then he walked away. He didn't have time to listen to something he wasn't going to do. He knew people meant well, but when someone insisted, it made him angry. It almost felt like they were trying to pull him away from his son.

A social worker approached Rebecca and Scott to say she had gotten them a room at the Ronald McDonald House. It was just down the block. The Batesons thanked the woman, but said they didn't need it. Checking into an inn-like setting seemed indulgent and trivial. And a block away? Rebecca felt it might as well be in Egypt. The social worker said the room would remain theirs. She handed Rebecca a key. "Use it," she said. "Take a shower, relax."

Rebecca decided it was at least a place to put gifts that had piled up in the family room. She took an armload of things and walked there. It was a lovely room. That made her uncomfortable. She felt guilty lingering in so pleasant an escape. She could not imagine sleeping there. Something else about it made her uncomfortable. Perhaps it was unfair, but to Rebecca, a room in the Ronald McDonald House meant her son was terminally ill. She dropped the gifts and quickly returned to the pediatric intensive care unit.

Rebecca began to read to Andrew. She often picked a book called *I Love You This Much.* It had a rabbit on the cover, and reading it became a nightly ritual. Rebecca sat in one of the vinyl chairs, high enough to be on Andrew's level. She read as if he were awake. It was never "I don't know whether he'll hear me." She just said, "Andrew, I'm going to read you a book, okay, hon?" Then she told him the name of it. As far as Rebecca was concerned, Andrew heard her.

Watching this gave Scott a small moment of peace. He felt that on some level Rebecca's voice was registering with Andrew. Had Scott been in that same place, a boy in the dark, the sound of his mother reading would have soothed him. As she read Scott could hear the whoosh of the respirator. He heard the rhythm of the pumps, each with its own cadence. He heard the heart monitor.

Staffers came in to check things, but Rebecca just kept reading. She only paused if nurses leaned over her.

"I'm sorry," Rebecca said, "do you need to get by?"

"No, no," the nurses always answered. "Make believe I'm not here."

The medical machinery kept going, but to Scott it was almost as if Andrew were home in his bed. Scott realized that's just where they had been the week before, reading this same book. Now they were here. Last week was a long time ago.

Rebecca looked out the window onto Interstate 95. The traffic mesmerized her. As night fell, the number of trucks grew. After 2 A.M., it was almost nothing but tractor-trailers. The morning commute started at 6:30 A.M., coming more to life with each minute. The sun rose beyond the head of Narragansett Bay in shades of orange and red. Midday, a crew started working the lanes of Route 95, so traffic backed up during evening rush hour. Rebecca felt that she qualified as an eye-in-the-sky—minus the helicopter.

She didn't notice too much on the bay; it was the interstate that caught her eye. She watched the cars as if they were fish in an aquarium. Often she spotted rescue vehicles a mile or so away and tracked them to Hasbro itself, or the other hospitals nearby. Sometimes she clocked how long they took. She wondered what was going on inside, and who it might be.

Rebecca took special notice of cars with luggage carriers on the roof. She pictured families on vacation and wondered where they were going. She imagined her own family in such a car right then, healthy and on their way. She imagined that those heading north were going to the mountains, and those traveling south were going to the beach. She never thought they were coming home. She always pictured them on their way.

The Batesons had been due to leave for the mountains on Saturday, July 5, the day after Andrew entered the hospital. They and some friends had rented a condominium for a week in Waterville Valley,

New Hampshire. It was going to be their big summer escape. They would ride the gondola at Wildcat and the alpine slide at Attitash and swim in the lakes. Of course they would go to Story Land. Growing up, Rebecca had gone there every year with her family, all the uncles and aunts and cousins. She visualized the nursery rhyme themes. You could spend a whole day there. She loved that part of New England. Some people found peace at the ocean, but for her it was the mountains.

Sitting in the hospital room, she let her thoughts go to the condominium itself, which they had rented before. It was all light and glass. Around it, there was the smell of natural pine. Had they been there now, Rebecca would have sat outside each morning to have her coffee. There would be no monitor or pump sounds, just the breeze through pine trees. That was what she thought of as she gazed down at the cars with the luggage carriers on top.

Rebecca was an observant Catholic, but wouldn't describe herself as overly religious. Going to Mass once a week was enough. At least she usually went once a week.

Before this happened, Rebecca had a deal going with God. She wouldn't ask for lots of money and big houses, and would make sure to thank Him every day for what He had given her. In return, she asked only that He keep things on an even keel; just don't give her more than she could handle. She felt now that He had let down His end of the bargain. It struck her as unfair. Nevertheless, she did not stop praying. Lately, it was about Andrew's hands. "God," she prayed, "if You have to take anything, take his feet." Then she got angry at having to barter that way. This was not a conversation she should be having with God. Why would He do this to a child? But please, take his feet if You have to. Then she asked Him please not to let Andrew die.

Rebecca and Andrew used to have a daily ritual. She had him extend his hands, palms up. Then she would touch one finger at a time, reciting the five main rules. The first three were no playing with matches, no crossing the street, and no touching gasoline, which meant anything under the kitchen sink. No talking to strangers was the fourth rule. His pinkie was the last: "No coming into Mom and Dad's bed." Andrew used to do that all the time. They would wake at 3 A.M. and he would be standing there.

"Andrew, what are you doing?"

"I want to come in with you guys."

For all they knew, he had been there twenty minutes. Some mornings they found him curled on the floor of their room. Erin never did that, but Andrew was a regular. So that became the fifth rule. Don't come into Mommy and Daddy's bed. In the hospital, Rebecca decided to resume the rule ritual. Each night she counted on his swollen fingertips, speaking aloud. No playing with matches, no crossing the street, no touching gasoline, no talking to strangers. She decided to change the last one. She touched his pinkie and said, "I love you." If he ever wanted to come into their bed again, that would be fine. She probably should have changed the rule long ago, since it never worked anyway.

Dr. Kleinman examined Andrew's fingers. His whole hands were swollen and dark. Scott asked Dr. Kleinman what she thought.

"They still look dusky to me," she said. That word came up often.

Kleinman said there were signs that a little bit of good blood was working past the clotting here and there, but the fingers remained troubling.

By this sixth day, most of the toes were black. Scott could no longer deny that. The circulation had apparently stopped, or nearly so. That was why the fingers scared him. The way they looked now was how Andrew's toes had looked a few days before.

Casey Little and Lori LaFrance were therapists in Hasbro's rehabilitation department. They were asked to begin working with Andrew's hands and legs. They gowned up and went into his room. They had treated few patients so restricted by medical attachments.

Andrew had a lot onboard. Too much, really. They and the team decided it was too early.

The two began regularly checking on him. They would not have been surprised had his name been gone from the door; the day-to-day was that pessimistic.

Soon they decided it was important to try some work. Although Andrew was in a coma, Casey introduced herself to him. "I'm the occupational therapist," she said. "I'm just going to move your fingers a little so your joints don't get stiff."

Lori LaFrance saw the photographs of Andrew playing baseball. "It's kind of like warming up before a game," Lori said to him. "Like stretching before you play."

The dressings on Andrew's hands made therapy difficult. The bandaging reminded Casey of boxing gloves, which felt appropriate to her, given how hard he was fighting. More than once, as they ranged Andrew's fingers, Lori saw tears run down his cheeks. That was a hard sight. She held it together until she got back to the office, then broke down a little.

Every morning a nurse pushed on each fingernail to see how fast the blood came back. That exam got Scott's attention, and he began to do it himself. He pressed Andrew's nails and counted. "Come on," he said to himself, "come back fast. Please come back fast." It seldom did. It took four seconds or more. It should have taken a half second or less. He repeated the test throughout the day.

Sometimes Scott just stared at Andrew's fingers, trying to will them to be lighter. Then he caught himself; maybe he was staring so much he had lost perspective. He asked the nurses what they thought. Were Andrew's fingers different? Better?

"They still look a little dusky." Scott learned to read the nurses' tone. They could give the same answer two days in a row, but the way they said it told him if things were worse.

The darker the fingers got, the more Scott negotiated with God. If You have to take something, he prayed, take *my* legs. Take *my* feet. Why take his? He's six. I'm forty-five.

Sometimes Scott got angry. "What's the deal here," he said to God in a prayer. "How can You take his feet and hands, too?" That was more than any person should have to pay, especially a six-year-old boy. He would send up such thoughts as he sat by Andrew.

The chapel was directly below the family room. Scott began to go there often. Usually it was just him, or one other person. He knelt, folded his hands, and asked God please to come down and help his son get better. Andrew was young; it couldn't be time for him to go yet.

In the past, Scott had not been big on prayer, except before sleep, when he'd briefly ask God to keep his family safe. When he thought back to that, it made him angry. God had broken his trust. *I prayed every night to keep my children all right,* he thought, *and here we are.* Perhaps this wasn't God's intention. But the thing was, why couldn't He stop it? That was Scott's question all the time.

Occasionally, God did feel close by. The more intensely Scott prayed, the more he sensed that closeness. It was hard to explain that to people, so he seldom tried. It was just a feeling that God heard him, and was going to help. The chapel became a comfortable place for him.

One morning the Batesons left together for the cafeteria, passing the chapel on the way. Scott said he would like to go in for a moment. Rebecca said she would wait. She was in no hurry. Often, eating made her feel guilty, even ill. After a few minutes, she felt silly standing in the corridor, so she walked in. She sat apart from Scott and tried praying. She tried for ten minutes but wasn't able to find comfort there. She was still angry at God. She went back out to the hallway.

Dr. Kleinman called in a burn surgeon to examine Andrew's wounds. He was described as a brilliant man at the top of his field nationally.

When he was done consulting with Kleinman, he asked the Batesons if he could speak with them.

Rebecca and Scott went with him to the consultation room. He sat in one chair, Rebecca in another, Scott on the couch. It was about 6 P.M. They had been in the hospital almost a week. The Batesons were taken aback at how the conversation began.

"Your son's skin is the least of his problems," the doctor said. "This kid's on dialysis, a ventilator. He's being kept alive."

He talked a bit about Andrew's skin wounds, then said, "This is nothing that you'll ever have to worry about, because I don't think your son's going to survive."

Rebecca could not stop herself. "Where have you been for the last six days?" she said. "Don't you dare come in here and tell me to give up on my son, because I'm not going to do it."

"Your son's on dialysis," the doctor said. "He can't even keep his blood pressure. Or heart rate. I think you're being seriously misled."

"You were not called in here to talk about his kidneys, or his heart," Rebecca said. "You were called in to talk about his skin. If you don't have anything to say about Andrew's skin, this conversation is over."

The doctor kept talking. Look at Andrew's circulation, he said; look at his hands, his legs. He's seriously ill. The doctor had almost no hope that their son would pull through.

Rebecca felt as though her head would explode. So much had been done on Andrew's behalf, and now this burn surgeon was dismissing the whole effort. As far as he was concerned, it was a waste of time. He was so blunt and sure of himself as to make her wonder about the other doctors. Scott sat there dumbfounded. The doctor tried to continue, but Rebecca interrupted.

"I said, this conversation is over."

He started out the door. "I think I need to have a talk with Dr. Kleinman," he said, and was gone.

Deb Powers was in the corridor when her younger sister

emerged from the sit-down. Scott went in one direction, Rebecca in another. Deb caught up to her. Rebecca told her what had been said.

Deb thought: *We've all tried hard to keep up hope, and in one minute, this son of a bitch wiped that out. It was as if he'd said everyone had lied to the family.*

The pediatric ICU was a small place, and people began to hear about the encounter. Soon Dr. Kleinman sought out Rebecca. "I am so sorry that happened," Kleinman said. "You have to believe me. Yes, your son is critically ill, but we're going to do everything to help him survive this."

"I don't want him anywhere near my son again," Rebecca said of the burn specialist. "I don't care if he's the expert; I need people who are looking out for Andrew's best interest."

Rebecca had to walk this off. She headed to the outdoor garden behind the hospital. She had been there several times before. Usually it made her feel far away. It did not have that effect at the moment.

Family members joined her. "Is he right and everybody else wrong?" Rebecca asked. Her sister Deb said Dr. Kleinman had gotten Andrew through the first days; she would get him through the next ones, too. Others tried to reassure Rebecca, but she was not able to listen. She was furious, not just at the burn surgeon, but at everything.

Then she began to cry. "Why did this happen to us?" she said. "Why did this happen to my son?" Everyone had tried to stay positive, she thought, and now this clown was saying it was all for nothing. She felt that if she could hurt that man, she would. And then she didn't care about him; all she cared about was Andrew, and she could not stop crying.

Chapter 5

"Let him be the boy that he was . . ."

At first the family waiting room seemed big to Deb Powers. But each day it got smaller. Sometimes, there were fifteen people there for Andrew. At one point, some friends showed up with a cooler so huge that two people had to lug it. It was full of home-cooked meals. That was pretty much how it went. Rebecca and Scott hoped that Andrew, though unconscious, would sense the presence of those who knew him, and draw from it.

Lynn Cavaliero was the manager of the pediatric ICU. She worked closely with Suzanne Kiniry, clinical nurse specialist. The two were impressed by the number of folks who came for this child. They had seldom, if ever, seen so many callers. To Lynn, they weren't typical hospital stops; people stayed three or four hours. Some came at midnight. Technically, Hasbro had visiting times, but in the intensive care unit they weren't enforced. The nurses let it go.

Andrew's sister, Erin, slept either at her aunt Jen's or the Mullens' across the street. It was a load off Scott and Rebecca's minds. People took care of their house, too. It allowed the Batesons never to leave the hospital. Lynn Cavaliero, the PICU manager, didn't feel it was luck that the parents had such support. It told her something about them.

· · ·

One night, Rhonda Mullen called Rebecca at eleven. Erin's asthma was acting up, and she'd left her nebulizer at her aunt Jen's, a half hour away. Two of Andrew's older cousins, Sean Costello and Scott Powers, had just gotten to Hasbro. Both were twenty-something years old.

"We'll go," one said.

All that way? They wouldn't be home until well past midnight. Were they sure?

They were. They headed to the parking lot. At 12:30 A.M., the two reappeared at the hospital, errand done. Rebecca asked why they hadn't just gone home to bed.

Because they hadn't gotten their visit in, they said. They stayed until two. That's how it went.

Scott worked in quality control at Foremost Printers. He did not call in that first week since he had it off for vacation. Rebecca's sister Janice called for him. The owner said Scott shouldn't worry. He should take as long as he needed. Scott was surprised when his checks kept coming. He could see them giving him time, but paying him? That was above what Scott would have thought. Later he learned that his co-workers had donated vacation days to keep him beside Andrew. They also took up a collection to help with the mortgage.

Rebecca's sisters worried about her physically. She was losing weight. So was Scott. "Andrew needs you," Deb said. "You have to keep up your stamina. At least have a doughnut." Eating, Rebecca said, made her feel ill. It felt like food just sat in her throat. Except for coffee, she couldn't swallow much.

The sisters kept pushing her about sleep. She wouldn't be any good to anyone if she didn't get rest. They said there were couches in the family room—only yards away from Andrew.

"I can't leave him," she said. What if he woke up with only strangers around?

"One of us will be there," said Jennifer.

...

Rebecca had asked whether other children with this bad a case had lived. The nurses mentioned a little boy named Giovanni, from nearby Fall River, Massachusetts. Rebecca asked about meeting his family. They came to the PICU a few days later, after physical therapy downstairs. The mom had brought some of his older brothers and sisters, who scattered, except for one who sat protectively near Giovanni. She also brought photographs of her son covered with purpura welts.

At first, the mother said, they thought Giovanni would lose only his toes. He ended up losing a leg above the knee. Giovanni seemed the same age as Andrew. He was in a wheelchair. He hadn't gotten a prosthetic leg yet, and wore a pair of shorts. It wasn't something you see very often. It sort of took Rebecca's breath away.

At one point Giovanni started horsing around with his brother, but most of the time he was withdrawn and shy. Rebecca wondered if that was his personality or the effect of the illness.

Giovanni's shyness worried Scott, too. Andrew had never been the quiet kind. Would he end up that way? Scott didn't ask about Giovanni's leg. The whole matter of amputation and wheelchairs was jarring to him. He wasn't ready to look at that yet.

Until now, the matter of Scott's car had slipped his mind. Suddenly, something made him remember it. He had left it outside the emergency room. He mentioned it to one of the staff. They told him not to worry, they would make sure security knew. It had been parked in a fifteen-minute space. It was now a week later.

By this point, Andrew's toes had turned almost black. It was hard for Scott to deny what was happening. He told God he would let the toes go, as long as Andrew still had a foot and ankle. Then Andrew's ankle pulses began getting weaker.

As Andrew's extremities worsened, Scott became more withdrawn. Sometimes if he saw visitors in the family room, he'd quickly say hello, then continue down the hall. He didn't want to be around the whole crowd, being asked yet again how Andrew was doing. He was polite if people came up to him, but he preferred retreating somewhere. He felt like he was in a dark, separate place, and needed to be there.

Scott was in the family room when he noticed Erin reaching for a can of Coke. There were often sodas sitting around.

"Is that yours?" Scott asked his daughter. His brother George was there. He could tell Scott was tense.

Yes, said Erin, it was hers.

"Are you sure?" Scott asked. Then he said he wasn't taking any chances, not for a lousy seventy-five-cent soda, and threw it in the wastebasket.

Everyone, including Rebecca, just looked at him.

Mike Day, the Batesons' across-the-street neighbor, became a regular at night, often staying until 3 or 4 A.M. Andrew was touch-and-go, and Mike thought somebody should be around. As a Providence fireman, Mike was used to a few hours' sleep. Mike wasn't a big talker, but he was a good friend. He understood how to just be there.

One night he was sitting alone with Scott, just the two of them. For a while, neither spoke.

Finally, Mike said, "I got a new laptop."

He had brought it with him. He knew Scott was into computers. Mike opened it up to show him.

"I picked it up real cheap," said Mike.

"What's it got?" Scott asked.

"It's a 486." It didn't have a CD drive, which kept the weight off. But it did have a detachable three-and-a-half. They talked about its other features for a bit. Mike felt that changing the subject was good for Scott.

Mike was comfortable letting silences fall. Sometimes that got Scott to open up. He'd withdraw if pressed, but let him alone long enough and he might come around. One night, Scott turned to Mike and asked what would happen if Andrew lost his feet or hands.

No one knew about that yet, Mike said.

"What if he can't walk?" Scott said.

"He's a kid," Mike said. "Kids are resilient."

But what, Scott asked, if people don't think he's normal? He didn't understand why all this was happening.

Mike said he didn't either.

Scott's thoughts retreated inside, and he grew quiet. Mike picked up that Scott didn't want to talk about it anymore. He could relate. Often, Mike thought, that's how men deal with hard things—by pulling in.

Rebecca and her sisters felt it important to have positive news. They came up with what they called a happy list. It would give Rebecca things to hold on to each day. The nurses put together the first one on a paper towel. It was a stretch to find positives. Creatinine levels were lower. Also, they'd cut back on Andrew's dopamine. That was about it.

Sometimes when Rebecca and Scott talked to Andrew, his eyelids fluttered. The nurses said it could be a sign that Andrew was hearing them. As a test, Rebecca asked from time to time if he wanted her in the room with him. Once Andrew nodded. That heartened her. She tried to tell herself it was a moment of connection. But she admitted it was probably just coincidence.

Rebecca told visitors that if they were in the room, they were not just sitting there; she wanted them talking to her son. It wasn't easy having a conversation with an unconscious child, so at times the aunts got a little nutty about it. Janice Costello would poke fun at Andrew, sing to him, sometimes even dance.

The uncles tended to make offers. Deb's husband, Steve, said he wanted to see the movie *George of the Jungle*, but would wait until he could take Andrew. One of Scott's brothers promised to take him to Monster Trucks.

"Andrew," Deb said at one point, "when you wake up, Uncle Steve here is going to put a Speedo on and do cartwheels down the corridor." That would have been a sight, as Uncle Steve was quite heavy.

Two weeks before Andrew fell sick, his cousin Beth had gotten engaged. The date wasn't for a year, but she was already talking about plans.

"Andrew will dance at my wedding," Beth told people at the hospital. "And you're going to wear a tuxedo," she told Andrew as he lay there unconscious, "whether you like it or not."

Maureen Pinksaw put on a mask and went into the room. She had been Andrew's kindergarten teacher at the Robert F. Kennedy School in Providence. Rebecca stood and asked her to sit by Andrew. He was discolored and swollen.

"It's all right," Rebecca said, "you can touch him."

Mrs. Pinksaw held Andrew's arm. The respirator breathed for him. "I've got some chocolate-chip cookies for a snack," she told him.

Mrs. Pinksaw was forty-one and wouldn't have traded teaching kindergarten for any other job. By year's end, everyone was a big happy family. She had graduated Andrew a month before. It was hard to see him amid all these machines. Something made her think of the previous May, when the class had put on a circus.

"Andrew," she said to him, "do you remember being a lion?" He had played the part with a lot of gusto. "Remember A.J. and Curtis and Nicholas? Remember the schoolyard? How you tried to scare the girls?"

Mrs. Pinksaw began visiting twice a week, driving forty minutes from her home near Newport. "The teacher's here," people told the Batesons. Rebecca and Scott usually excused themselves, saying they were going to the cafeteria. They wanted Andrew to have Mrs. Pinksaw to himself. At one point Scott said to her, "... if he lives." That "if" was a real hard word for Mrs. Pinksaw.

She decided to buy a musical tape called *Close Your Eyes* for Andrew. They had used it in class, playing various cuts to signal it being time to move to the next activity, an old kindergarten trick. Mrs. Pinksaw would also bring a bag of books. She sat by Andrew's bed, took one out, and began to read the same way as in class, using different voices for the characters.

She usually picked *Miss Nelson Is Missing,* one of Mrs. Pinksaw's favorites. Miss Nelson was a very nice teacher whose students didn't treat her well. They threw spitballs and such. One day the school sent in a substitute, Miss Viola Swamp. She was much stricter than Miss Nelson. She made them sit up, be quiet, work hard. She didn't talk to them pleasantly at all. When Miss Nelson came back, they finally appreciated her.

Now, as Andrew lay there, Mrs. Pinksaw put on her best Viola Swamp voice. That was easier in front of twenty-six kids than in a hospital room with nurses nearby. But Mrs. Pinksaw made herself do it.

Not to stereotype, but Mrs. Pinksaw found Andrew very boyish. He was into sports and had this thing about Harley-Davidson items. He used to wear a leather vest with leather fringe to class. It didn't bother him what anyone else thought. As Mrs. Pinksaw put it, he beat to his own drummer. Once Mrs. Pinksaw kidded him about it, asking if he was getting ready for an Indian feast. Andrew laughed, and said, "Yeah." He had quite a good sense of humor.

One thing you wouldn't call Andrew was shy. At year's end he volunteered to sing a solo at graduation. Before the ceremony, Rebecca asked Mrs. Pinksaw to please make sure his shirt was tucked in. Andrew wasn't exactly a jacket-and-tie person, so Mrs. Pinksaw did her best. By the time he was up there, his shirttail was out again. He didn't care for looking formal.

Andrew's only issue had been learning to let go of Mom each morning after drop-off. He didn't want her to leave. It had taken him over a month to get over that.

Scott and Rebecca were surprised when the kindergarten teacher's aides, Mrs. Winkleman and Mrs. Ryan, also visited the hospital. The school principal, Mrs. Koshgarian, came to visit Andrew too. The Batesons never knew who would be next. Mary St. Jacques, the emergency room nurse, came up daily. It wasn't like Mary to visit so often, but something about Andrew got to her. She figured it couldn't hurt to say a prayer before leaving, so she always did. She was sure the ICU nurses said a few too.

Father Joe Escobar kept the oil of the sick on his bedroom bureau. It was used to anoint people who were ill. He placed his car keys next to it. Perhaps once a month he was awakened by a phone call and had to quickly grab both. He also took a bottle of holy water, just in case. When people had already died, they could not be anointed. Instead, the body was blessed with holy water.

He became a regular visitor. Early on, when he brought out the metal oil stock, it startled Rebecca and Scott. The two were alarmed by anything that implied last rites. Father Joe explained that this was a healing ritual, not a preparation for death. When Rebecca still looked skeptical, Father Joe talked about Brian Feeney, a boy from St. Pius who had been hit by a car three years before while crossing a Providence street. Brian was ten and had suffered a brain injury. He was in a coma for three weeks. The doctors offered little hope that he would walk, speak, or have normal functions. But he woke before Christmas, now played Little League, and was doing well in school. The doctors didn't have a good explanation for Brian's recovery, but Father Joe told Rebecca he had anointed the boy shortly after the accident. He believed that had played some part.

Standing at Andrew's bedside, Father Joe began. "Lord, God, You have said to us through Your apostle James: 'Are there people sick among you?'"

Both nurses and machines continued their work. Father Joe placed a hand on Andrew's head and prayed silently. Then he spoke aloud: "Lord, You've told us that the sick upon whom we lay our hands will recover." He took out the oil, dipped his thumb in it, and made the sign of the cross on both Andrew's forehead and his palms. He had to be careful of the IVs and skin lesions. "Through this holy anointing, may the Lord in His love and mercy help you with the grace of the Holy Spirit."

Father Joe ended with a blessing asking healing for Andrew. "Give him strength in this illness, bless the doctors and nurses who care for him. Restore him. We ask this through Christ our Lord."

Father Joe often stayed with the Batesons for hours. He spoke of another time he had seen the healing capacity of anointing. He was called to baptize a baby boy named Daniel Murphy. Usually it was done when an infant was a month or two old, but this child had heart problems soon after birth and was to be taken to Boston for surgery. It was Father Joe's first emergency baptism. He had to ask an older priest for a quick refresher on how to do it. He grabbed his oils and was soon at the hospital. They took him to the special-care nursery. He remembered having seen the mother pregnant at the church. He bent over the child.

"I baptize you in the name of the Father and the Son and the Holy Spirit," he said.

Father Joe then chose to anoint the child, feeling that a prayer of healing could help. When the family got to Boston that night, the cardiogram was different than it had been in Providence. The doctors kept him under observation several days, then chose not to operate.

That was five years before. Though they continued to monitor him, the boy had never had surgery. "I believe it was healing," Father Joe told Scott and Rebecca of the anointing. "It happens. It's God's grace. It's nothing I do. I'm just there to say the words and offer the prayer."

Father Joe was a down-to-earth priest, prone toward kidding

his more serious colleagues. "He's so *spiritual*," he would quip. Or "He's such a *priest*." But he believed in prayer strongly enough to have given up the possibility of a wife and children in its name.

Both Father Joe and Father Ken came to the hospital daily. Scott thought they were both well spoken when they got to the ad-lib part of prayers. Priests, he thought, had a good way of saying things. He always felt something extra when they were in the room. He hoped it would get inside Andrew.

Scott and Rebecca were in the garden. Father Joe was nearby, giving them some space. By now Rebecca had grown concerned that she and her husband seldom talked anymore, at least in any depth. She decided, with Father Joe's presence making it safe, that she would reach out to Scott.

She told him they had a good marriage and foundation. That was more than she could say for many couples who weren't coping with a crisis. No matter what happened, she said, they had that foundation. It would help sustain the family.

Scott didn't respond. He didn't see the value of feel-good phrases like "It'll be fine." That was just talk. It wasn't real.

Rebecca didn't say any more. It was hard for her to reach out that way and not get anything back.

She began to share less and less with Scott, having picked up a "don't come near me" demeanor from him. Rebecca felt as though they were losing each other. She didn't mention these feelings to anyone, though, not even her sisters. That would have put it out there. Then she wouldn't be able to take it back.

Scott was not aware that Rebecca was pushing away from him. He wasn't looking for support right now, so he didn't miss it. Given what Andrew was facing, Scott felt it indulgent to seek sympathy for himself. As a man, that just didn't seem right to him. It was why he didn't respond when Rebecca had tried to offer comfort.

. . .

In the middle of the second week, Scott felt it might help to write in a diary. It was Wednesday, July 9. He sat down in a chair in the family room with a pen and notebook. He began to write.

"Woke up this morning . . ."

That was as far as he got. After a while he put the notebook away. He just wasn't able to get anything going.

Scott walked into the hospital chapel in early afternoon. Much of the front wall was stained glass of abstract design. The altar was a kind of podium, with room to kneel next to it. Scott took a seat toward the front. He was the only one there. After a few minutes he heard the door open. In came two young women, perhaps in their early twenties. They knelt to the right of the altar and said hello to him. Scott asked if they had someone in the hospital who was ill.

No. They were just there to pray.

They began doing so. They were quite vocal about it. They weren't screaming meemies or anything, but they prayed in a full tone, as if talking to someone. They were very intense, their hands clasped hard. They prayed like that for maybe ten minutes. It fascinated Scott. Then they stopped and looked at him. One asked if he was all right.

"No," he said. "No, I'm not. My six-year-old son is upstairs. He's contracted a disease and we're not sure if he's going to live."

They asked what had happened.

Well, his son's name was Andrew, and he had bacterial meningitis. He was hanging on for his life right now. He was in a coma.

The two asked if he wanted them to pray with him.

"Yes," Scott said. "Yes I would. Please do."

"When we pray," said one of the women, "we usually join hands. It makes it so it's a complete circle." Prayers, she said, were stronger when there was more than one person. They held hands and began.

At first Scott was uneasy. The women were almost trance-like. There could have been a war outside and they would have still been into this. It was like a spell or something. They certainly did pray with a lot of heart, though, asking that the Spirit come down and heal Andrew.

Scott was grateful for their emotion. He closed his eyes and joined in silently. If God hadn't heard him before, maybe He would hear Scott now. To be honest, it gave him chills down his back.

The two women slowed and stopped. One said she was sure God had heard them. They encouraged Scott to continue praying. They said God would listen to him when he prayed from the heart. As they were about to leave, he asked what brought them to the chapel.

"We were just nearby," one said. "We pray daily."

After they left, he sat there a few minutes, wondering how to think about it. Here were these two girls he didn't know from a hole in the wall. Why had they come there? Upstairs, he told Rebecca the story. He wondered to himself if it was a sign of one of those visits by an angel that people talk about. Of course, it was more likely just two women walking by who decided to pray. Probably that. It was hard to say.

A few days later, Scott was in the chapel when the two women came back in. It was Friday. They asked how Andrew had been doing. Would Scott like to pray again?

This time, one introduced herself as Andrea, the other as Angelica. The name of the second took Scott by surprise. He was far from some spiritual believer type, but it left him wondering. When he told Rebecca, she, too, thought it might be a sign.

Later they learned the girl worked at a hospital deli called Au Bon Pain. Still, that name meant something to both of them.

Lori Bateson was married to Scott's older brother Jimmy. She didn't think you could walk into Andrew's room without wanting to pray. At least she couldn't. She usually asked God to bring Andrew back to the family, even if he didn't have all his parts.

Uncle Jimmy, too, tried to face that there could be losses. "Let him be the boy that he was before he came into the hospital," Jimmy prayed. Jimmy tried to give the same message to Scott. As long as Andrew was still Andrew, he would say, it would work out.

John Lamberton was married to Scott's sister, Karen. He was a construction manager. He wasn't religious at all, not a bit, never bothered with Sunday services. But those priests, Father Ken and Father Joe, struck John as exceptional. The two almost made him want to go to church—not quite, but almost. Even John began to say a prayer when he visited. It wasn't anything formal; he just did his own thing. If asked, he preferred not discussing details. He didn't want to get into it, prayer being private. A few times he got choked up, which surprised John about himself, as he wasn't the kind to cry at all.

Across the street from the Batesons' house, Cindy Day's four children had long had a routine of praying every night, but she thought it had as much to do with stalling lights-out as with some wonderful relationship with God. The four kids would name all their aunts, uncles, relatives, friends, and neighbors. Then they moved on to a whole litany of whomever else needed a prayer at the moment.

Stephanie, the child Andrew's age, would start praying for her dolls.

All right, Cindy would say, let's wrap it up. Was Stephanie finished?

No, she had one more thing she had to pray for.

What?

Um, she had to think of it. But it was important.

Stephanie . . .

That's why Mike and Cindy didn't have them pray on their knees. It was hard enough getting four kids tucked into bed once, let alone twice.

This past week had been different. It was about Andrew and no one else. They prayed hard. The children felt that prayer was something they could do for him.

. . .

It seemed that everyone at St. Pius Church was praying for Andrew too. Cindy had seldom heard of so much prayer offered up for one person.

Her husband, Mike, the fireman, had been only somewhat into prayer. But now he got more serious. Whenever he had a moment, he would send one up.

Steve Powers, Deb's husband, was probably the least spiritual person he knew. It wasn't his thing, not even a little. But whenever he visited the hospital he became aware of something. You'd have to be stone, he thought, not to sense it. Even Steve started to pray—not that it was the most comfortable thing for him to do.

Jennifer Lusignon, one of Rebecca's sisters, began getting calls from strangers who said they wanted to pray for Andrew. Friends of friends of friends. Sometimes the phone rang as early as 6:30 A.M. and as late as midnight with people wanting details.

The callers would start with unfamiliar names. "I'm sorry," one said, "you don't know me. I live in Florida. I heard about Andrew."

"How did you get my number?"

Well, my friend So-and-So said she was praying for this little boy in Rhode Island, and now the person calling wanted to include him in her own prayer circle.

Father Ken once came in with a fax from the Midwest. *Our group is praying for Andrew,* it said. Scott never had known what a prayer chain was. He was getting an education. He felt that a strong message was being sent to the Man.

Chapter 6

"Andrew, can you open your eyes?"

cott was alone at Andrew's bedside when Cindy Day, their neighbor, gowned up and came in. It was about 10:30 P.M. Rebecca was in the family room, trying to sleep. Andrew was having an unsettled night. Although in a coma, he sometimes got restless. It made the monitors go crazy, and there seemed to be nothing you could do for him. It left the parents quite stressed.

After several hours, Andrew at last calmed. Cindy got ready to leave. Scott asked if she had a few minutes. Would she mind coming to the chapel with him?

Cindy turned to the bed. "I'll see you later, Andrew. God bless you."

They took the elevator down a floor and walked to the front of the chapel. They knelt and prayed. Then they sat down on one of the benches. Scott told Cindy about the two women. He felt it was some kind of message.

Then he talked about Andrew's legs and hands. They remained in bad shape. Scott had a lot of fears about it.

No matter what happened, Cindy said, Andrew would bounce back. "Look at the type of kid he is. Nothing'll keep him down."

"Yeah," said Scott. "I hope you're right."

They prayed and talked some more. At times Scott got angry about what had happened. At other times he was confused by it.

They stayed in the chapel for about two hours. More than once Scott wept. They both did.

On another night Cindy was sitting with Rebecca in the family room. The two were alone. Rebecca had tried to sleep, but wasn't able to.

"Hard night, Bec?"

Nighttime usually was, Rebecca said. It was difficult for her to be alone with her thoughts. She would start to wonder "What if": What if he didn't come out of the coma? Or they had to take his legs above the knees? Or his hands? Or both? Would other kids treat him differently? Would they still like him if he couldn't keep up?

It wasn't going to change who he was, Cindy Day said. The kids on the block would treat him like Andrew, as they always had.

Rebecca didn't seem convinced. What if this affected his brain? Left him less than he was?

Cindy said that Andrew's spirit, God bless him, would get him through.

They talked into the early hours.

Cindy often stayed in the hospital until Rebecca was asleep. Then she gathered her things and headed out. As she left she often sent up a prayer for the parents: "Please, God, give them the rest and strength they need." She said prayers for Andrew, too, but Cindy figured he was covered. She wanted to make sure Scott and Rebecca were taken care of, as well.

Cindy Day had four children, five if you counted Andrew, whom she sometimes referred to as "one of ours." Her youngest, Stephanie, was born weeks after Andrew in February of 1991. At times the mothers had them in the same crib. The whole street was close. You never knew whether you'd find the kids at the Days', the Batesons', or the Mullens'. Whichever house they went to, they pretty much belonged.

Cindy found it a very 1950s neighborhood. If the children weren't on bikes or Rollerblades, they were playing manhunt. Manhunt was like hide-and-seek, only more complicated. Few parents understood the rules. As it got dark, the moms and dads started calling them in, but it was always "We can't—we're playing manhunt."

Sometimes the girls staged shows on the lawns, complete with costumes. Often, Andrew was in there with them. He got a kick out of dressing up and being onstage—especially the onstage part.

Most of the kids Andrew's age were girls, but he liked hanging with older boys like Michael Day, Rory Madden, and Joseph Mullen. If they were wrestling, Andrew piled on. If it was karate, Andrew gave it a shot. Although they were elevenish and he was six, he was never shy about it.

If he got hurt, he wasn't always gracious. "You did that on purpose," Andrew said.

Come on, Andrew, it was an accident.

"I'm not going to be your friend anymore," he'd say, and run home. Five minutes later, he was always back.

They liked to skateboard down the block's steepest driveway, flying into the street. The parents ended up standing there, yelling for cars to slow down. That was easier than trying to get the kids to stop. Especially Andrew. God forbid, thought Cindy Day, you ever told him he couldn't do something.

Often Rebecca got exasperated with him. She would call across the street for him to come home for dinner.

"Okay," Andrew would yell from Mike and Cindy Day's front yard.

Ten minutes later Rebecca would call again. No response. Most kids had selective hearing, but Mike Day found Andrew's especially well developed. He could tune his parents right out.

When forced to come home, he didn't make it easy. Sometimes he threw what Mike Day called an Andrew-tantrum. He didn't kick and scream, but he could toss out a lot of "no's" and "I don't want to's." Mike was amused by it. It was nice for it to be somebody else's kid for a change.

Those "no's" could really irk Rebecca. At such times she asked Cindy Day, "Is it ever going to get better?"

"It'll come," Cindy said.

"He doesn't do anything I want him to do."

It's not really defiance, Cindy said; Andrew just had a lot of spirit.

It wasn't always easy for Rebecca to see the difference.

Once Andrew walked into the Days' house while Mike was straightening things up. He stood next to Mike for a few seconds, then said, "What are you doing?" Andrew wasn't shy about asking an adult anything.

Cleaning, said Mike.

"Why?"

Because my wife wants me to.

"Yeah? How come?"

Because she'll be upset if I don't.

"Why?"

Because she wants the house clean.

"Why does she?"

Mike never knew a kid to ask so many questions.

One morning, Mike began caulking the foundation. Soon, there was Andrew.

"What are you doing?"

I'm filling the cracks, said Mike.

"Why?"

So the draft won't get in.

"Why you doing it now?"

I've got to get it done before the winter.

"What's that stuff?"

Caulking.

"What's it made of?"

It's made to fill the spaces.

"Why are you doing it?"

So the draft won't get in.

"Can I try?"

If Mike called his kids in for the night, Andrew usually questioned him about that, too.

"What are you doing?" Andrew asked.

It's bedtime, Andrew.

"Already?"

I'm afraid so.

Without missing a beat, Andrew would ask: "Can they sleep over?"

Same thing whenever Andrew saw the Days putting their kids in the car. It was always "Can I come too?"

Maria Amaral was one of Rebecca's oldest friends. The Batesons had planned their New Hampshire vacation with Maria and her husband, Manny, the week Andrew went into the hospital. Rebecca and Scott insisted the Amarals use the condo without them. The Amarals drove up and did their best, but they returned after four days. That evening, Maria Amaral went to the hospital. Several times, as she looked on, the nurses had to stabilize Andrew. On later visits, there always seemed to be a bedside crisis of one kind or another: Andrew's legs, his fingers, the burns. She noticed that Andrew's hands had become clawlike, in the way of long-term coma patients.

Growing up in the blue-collar town of West Warwick, Maria and Rebecca had gone through the whole 7th and 8th grade thing together: sleepovers, hairdos, boyfriends. They were bridesmaids at each other's weddings. They each had two children, close to the same ages. The two couples went out together often and tried to vacation together, too.

When Andrew wanted something, Maria felt that not much stood in his way. That was his personality in a nutshell: "One more time."

It got to Rebecca. "He tries me so much," she told Maria.

For example, he would always be asking for one more cookie. "Andrew," Rebecca said, "we're about to have dinner."

"But Mom, Mom—just one more."

Not right now, honey.

"Just one, Mom . . ."

Persistence, said Maria, wasn't a bad trait. It could get Andrew far. Rebecca considered it small comfort.

The two friends sat down in the hospital consultation room.

"Becca," Maria said, "how you feeling?"

Rebecca told her she was hoping for a miracle. Then she said she'd be grateful just to have Andrew alive.

Maria said that even if the worst happened to his legs Andrew would not be slowed down. He'd still ride a bike. Knowing Andrew, Maria really believed it.

Maria thought, *What kind of bacteria is this, that can start after bedtime and kill a child before he wakes?*

At night she began to check her children for rashes. Then she set her alarm for 3 A.M. and checked them again. When she got up at dawn, she did a third check. From time to time Maria dreamed about it. In one of the dreams, she saw her son Shane, who was nine, without legs. In another, Maria saw him covered with those black spots. When she woke up, she went into Shane's room to make sure she had only dreamed it.

Rebecca asked her sisters to massage Andrew's feet when they were in the room. The doctors said it wouldn't do any good, but the sisters sensed that it did something for Rebecca, so they stayed at it, even when she wasn't there to see.

The four sisters had grown up close. They shared rooms and

they shared clothes. Their dad, Northeast circulation manager for the *National Enquirer*, was often on the road, and they'd joke that Rebecca, the youngest, ended up with three extra mothers.

The sisters could be hard on each other, but they were the only ones allowed to be that way. "I can trash my sister," Janice would joke, "but no one else can."

Their father used to say to his sons-in-law: "You didn't marry one of them; you married all four."

If one had an argument with her husband and it got around, another sister might say, "Bad enough you got your wife angry; now you got us angry too." The husbands were never sure if they were joking.

The sisters believed that of all the husbands, Scott faced the toughest hurdle, since he was marrying the baby. "He didn't just have to pass inspection with the parents," said Jen, "he had to pass inspection with us."

Early on, the brothers-in-law took Scott for a beer to warn him about what he was getting into. They repeated the line about marrying not one, but all four. Scott said he understood.

Each sister had a holiday or two. Janice Costello had Thanksgiving and Easter. Deb Powers had Christmas. Labor Day was Jennifer's, and so was July Fourth. That gathering usually started at noon and ended at midnight. They swam, played basketball, and pitched horseshoes. All holidays were big, but July Fourth was especially so. There were usually over fifty people at the Costellos'. That was a lot of phone calls to make when they heard Andrew was sick and needed to cancel.

A week or so after Andrew got sick, Rebecca's sister Jennifer brought something for her to sleep in. It was a conservative nightgown, but the brand was Victoria's Secret.

"I don't think so," Rebecca said. "Floating around the ICU in lingerie while my son is lying there?"

Instead, she slept in regular clothes, usually a sweatsuit, especially when Andrew had a fever. The temperature in his room was kept low then, leaving Rebecca chilled.

Rebecca's sisters told her they were sick of the sundress she had been wearing for days. It was white with little blue flowers on it. They told her they were going to burn it so they'd never have to see it again. It made Rebecca realize how little attention she was paying to things that used to matter a lot to her.

Rebecca's sisters began to see a side of her they hadn't known. At meetings with doctors, she began to take charge, asking most of the questions. That was how she coped, focusing not on what had happened, but on what they could do about it.

Andrew's aunt Janice was there once when Andrew seemed to grow agitated. The young resident on duty prescribed Tylenol rather than sedatives.

"I think you need to give him something stronger," Rebecca said. "The Tylenol isn't cutting it."

The resident told her not to worry. "He doesn't feel anything. He's too heavily sedated."

"This is not fair to him," Rebecca said. "This is not fair to us. I'm his mother. I know."

The doctor relented, though not happily.

The nurses were different; they talked to Andrew as if he were awake. "Okay, hon," they said. "We're going to roll you over." They seemed to feel that at some level he could hear.

"You're in the hospital," they told him. "We're trying to help you get better. Try to rest now."

From time to time, the nurses gave Andrew an extra-big ventilator breath. The way they saw it, had they been the ones lying there, they'd have wanted one.

Janice Costello identified the nurses by sets of eyes, the only feature unobstructed by masks. Claire Piette's eyes were as blue as eyes got. "Angel eyes," Janice called them.

Often the nurses turned on the television. Better for Andrew to listen to cartoons, they thought, than people discussing whether his legs could be saved. Several told Rebecca about kids in comas who, after waking, remembered things they had heard while under. Those kinds of stories, the nurses said, changed the way they acted.

Claire Piette had heard doctors refer to PICU nurses as mother bears. She might not have argued with that. Some stayed hours after their shifts, not wanting to leave until everything was right. It was hard to explain why you developed such bonds with unconscious patients. It had to do with spending eight hours straight at their bedsides. Only other nurses, Claire thought, would understand.

Some doctors were as caring, but not all; at least that was how the sisters saw it. Jennifer Lusignon got aggravated when residents talked clinically in front of Andrew, as if he were just a case rather than a little boy.

"If you're in here," she told them, "you do not talk among yourselves about what's going on. Not about his condition, anyway."

The doctors said she didn't understand; the child was in a coma.

"Would you just mind taking that outside?" Jen responded.

The doctors did, though they looked at her as if she were odd.

Steve Powers, Rebecca's brother-in-law, had a name for the younger residents and interns. He referred to them as "sneakers." A real doctor, he thought, wore shoes. The residents wore sneakers. That put Steve off. He didn't appreciate doctors who presented themselves as kids. At times, he thought, a few acted the part. Here were doctors barely out of school who seemed to want to impress everyone. Adjust this, adjust that. He was there once when Claire Piette declined.

"No," she said. Just that: No. The issue was reducing the level of Andrew's painkillers. The young doctor was taken aback.

"But that's what I want you to do," he said.

Steve was enjoying this.

"I don't think that's a good idea," Claire said.

The doctor told her he expected her to do as asked.

She pleasantly suggested they call Dr. Kleinman. If the attending agreed, Claire said, she would do it. The resident grew red-faced and left the room. The nurses, Steve thought, knew what was going on. When they took a stand, they had a reason.

Dr. Kleinman had no problem with PICU nurses occasionally saying no to a resident. Usually they were right. It was easy, Kleinman thought, for physicians to step away, catch their breath, or make a phone call; intensive-care nurses didn't have that luxury. They had to stay at the bedside. They tracked everything and saw everything. In Kleinman's view, an experienced ICU nurse probably knew more about critical care than a resident.

Most of the disagreements were about sedation. Some residents felt it should be reduced, as did some intensivists. The PICU nurses, on the other hand, seldom pushed for lowered sedatives. Claire never did. Children attached to that much equipment, she believed, should be kept deep under. Andrew had a breathing tube in, lines in, and a kidney circuit; she didn't think a six-year-old should be aware of all that. Were it her child, she would not want him to know what was going on.

That's why she sometimes spoke up. Claire thought a PICU nurse shouldn't hold her tongue for fear someone might judge her impertinent. In her view, a nurse who did should perhaps look for work elsewhere. In sixteen years, Claire had never been tempted to change jobs. She believed this was what she was meant to do.

Andrew tended to grow unsettled around 7 P.M. One night was particularly bad. He wouldn't stop moving. His head went side to side, his legs up and down. He arched his back. The parents tried rubbing his stomach. "It's okay, Andrew," said Rebecca. "Mommy and Daddy are right here." Scott stroked his hair. They had done that so much Rebecca thought it would never lie forward again.

He remained unsettled, appearing as though in pain. The

nurses suggested they try turning him on his side. It took a while to do, given all the tubes and equipment. They braced him with rolled-up blankets. But it made things worse. Andrew struggled even more, so they turned him onto his back again. He continued to arch.

During the previous hours, they had reduced his sedation. Rebecca wondered if that left him just conscious enough to be aware of such discomforts as the vent, not to mention the weeks in one position. They reached under him to rub his back, then his legs. Finally, at around 9 P.M., he quieted. It took two hours of hard work. Rebecca and Scott were both drained.

At that point, a respiratory therapist came in. He wanted to suction Andrew's breathing tube. That sometimes left him restless. Scott thought: *Does he really have to do this right now? We just got him quieted down.* Scott didn't object, though. He figured the hospital had its routines.

There was one nurse in the room, an Asian woman, low-key and soft-spoken, a very nice lady. "There's no way you're doing anything to this child," she said.

It was just a suctioning, the therapist said.

"Not now. We just got him calmed down."

The therapist was sorry, but he needed to.

The nurse stood her ground. "You're not touching him."

Scott felt it was a little tense. She wasn't suggesting; she was telling him.

The therapist said he needed to do it now.

"You're not going to."

It was a standoff for a moment.

Finally, he backed down.

It occurred to Rebecca that she hadn't yet seen an ICU nurse intimidated by other staff, including doctors. If they didn't like something, they said so. They looked out for the patients.

A plastic surgeon came in to assess Andrew's wounds. Everyone was gowned and gloved, but he walked right in without precautions. Rebecca didn't like him right away. He seemed to feel he was God's gift. As he approached Andrew, a nurse stopped him.

"We're in precautions," she said.

"I'm not going to touch him," he said.

"At least wash your hands."

"Don't worry, I'm not going to touch him."

The nurse wouldn't budge.

"You have to go wash your hands."

He again said he wouldn't touch Andrew.

"Do you realize how easily this child could be infected?" she asked.

"But I won't—"

"I don't care," said the nurse. "Everybody washes their hands before you go near this child."

The plastic surgeon washed his hands.

Claire Piette preferred children as patients. Adults, she had found, tended to complain more. If a grown-up had a painful dressing change, he dwelled on it until the next one. On the other hand, you could do open-hearts on kids and they would be up in two days, playing Nintendo with their chest tubes in. Children did get scared about procedures, but once it was over they were on to the next thing. Adults, Claire thought, had a lot to learn from kids.

When Claire began nursing in the early 1980s, almost no one with advanced meningococcemia lived. The best the staff could do was prepare the parents. The nurses used to say, "They were happy and eating lunch, and dead by supper." It went that fast. What saved some children now wasn't antibiotics; they had always had those. It was technology—machines to support failed organs. That, and skills. Pediatric intensive care units had grown adept at resuscitating children in acute collapse. Claire felt Hasbro's team was among the most knowledgeable, given the practice they'd had over the past year. Nevertheless, she feared Andrew's condition might prove beyond them.

Claire remembered her first case. A little girl arrived looking normal except for a few small red dots. Six hours later she was black from lesions and swollen to twice her size from fluid infusions. No one, thought Claire, could prepare you for that sight. The child went into acute respiratory distress syndrome. Her lungs grew so soggy the ventilator could not push enough oxygen into her. When it was over, Claire was among those who had to tell the parents. Claire's home was a twenty-five-minute drive from the hospital. The trip was often her crying time back then. It still was.

Claire worked the second shift, three-forty-five to midnight. It allowed her to focus on her own four children by day. She sometimes prayed silently while she worked on Andrew. Usually she asked God to guide her hands. She was not a person who believed humans had direct life-and-death control; God acted through them. There was a greater power working overtime Up There, which Claire felt was only fair. As long as people were working hard down here, He might as well be too.

Spend enough years in the PICU, Claire thought, and you had to believe in that higher Something. She had seen cases where it was beyond medicine to save someone, yet the outcome was good. She was the charge nurse in December of 1995 when three little boys fell through the ice of Frog's Pond, a half hour from Providence. Claire took care of the one who was under the longest. He had been submerged thirty-seven minutes. He was ten years old. He had no heart rate when he came in, and every organ had failed. Brain scans showed no activity. He remained in a coma for two weeks. But he walked out of the hospital, apparently with no serious damage. The doctors could not explain it. That was the kind of thing that made Claire a believer.

Claire found it unusual in a case as severe as Andrew's that his lungs had not turned bad. If they had, he would almost certainly have died. That, too, made her wonder.

Dr. Kleinman was also surprised that Andrew had not developed acute respiratory distress syndrome. She found it remarkable. She did not necessarily ascribe it to exceptional care, but neither did she attribute it to faith. She thought they had simply gotten lucky. Sometimes that happened in medicine.

Michele Rozenberg began her nursing shift with a full-body assessment. "It's just Michele, Andrew. I'm going to examine you, make sure you're comfortable." She talked to all sedated patients, even comatose babies, so they wouldn't feel startled at the next touch.

"Andrew, can you open your eyes? I'm going to shine the light now." His pupils constricted well. That meant someone was still in there.

"Andrew, I'm just going to look into your mouth. I want to check your tube." His gums lined up correctly against the centimeter markings on the vent. To confirm it, she probed Andrew's throat for how the tube lay in his trachea. She checked his jugular veins. They were fine. Had they been distended, it could have meant heart congestion was backing blood into the great vessels of the neck. She inspected all lines, making sure the sites were clean and covered with sterile dressings. She moved on to the purpura welts. A few had opened. She would have to dress those. Every cracked wound had to be covered with Silvadene and gauze.

"I'm going to listen to your heart and lungs, Andrew."

The breathing tube created its own sounds, but Michele was able to distinguish those from the crackling she heard, a sign of mild fluid buildup in his chest. There were some decreased spaces, which told her the air wasn't reaching all the way. Still, his lungs seemed reasonably aerated. The bases had not collapsed. His breathing was in phase with the vent.

Michele told him she was going to suction his respirator tube. She put on an ambu bag, gave him three good breaths, detached the vent, quickly suctioned out the secretions, gave him a few more ambu breaths, and put him back on.

Next, his stomach. They kept a nasogastric tube inserted to evacuate air and digestive juices. There wasn't much of that, since the stomach shut down in IV-fed patients.

She shut off suction to listen for bowel sounds. Urine output was negligible because of kidney failure. She checked capillary re-fill, pressing his fingers and toes, then counting the seconds it took for the color to return. She got to eight, which was a disappointment. Despite meds to dilate his vessels, his hands and feet remained cold. He didn't seem to be perfusing.

Michele prepared to palpate his peripheral pulses. If she couldn't sense them by hand, she would have to use Doppler, which amplified so well you could hear not only pulsation, but blood flow. It sounded vaguely like running water. She checked the posterior popliteal pulses behind his knees, working around all the dressings. She continued distally, away from the center of the body, toward the feet. She checked the posterior tibial pulse behind the ankle, the pedal pulse atop the foot, and the anterior pulses as well. She had hoped to be able to palpate those, but she couldn't, and had to go to Doppler. Even with that, there was almost nothing. There wasn't much between the knee and the ankle, either. It did not look good for his extremities. Michele kept hoping, but it appeared very bleak.

Michele Rozenberg felt that caring for Andrew was like being on a moving treadmill. She stepped aboard as soon as she came on duty, and couldn't step off until her shift ended. Sometimes she had to ask a colleague to spell her while she collected herself in an empty room. This was usually after the stress of changing Andrew's skin dressings. Occasionally she saw tears come down his cheeks during the scrubbings. That got to her, and she needed to take a moment.

Nursing had given Michele Rozenberg a respect for children. Most remained brave through the worst ordeals. It was beyond what she herself would be able to do.

She had been lucky enough to meet Andrew before he went under. She could still picture him trying to reach out to his mom with his little arms. Michele had asked to remain one of Andrew's primary nurses, knowing that a familiar face can help a family. She thought back to her own baby. Ethan had been born four years before. He had been extremely premature, and did not survive. His primary nurses had been on duty from start to end, which had helped. They had come to know Ethan. That gave Michele comfort while her son was still alive.

When she came in each morning, Michele often found Scott or Rebecca in the big lounge chair by Andrew's bed. Neither seemed able to sleep soundly. Michele could tell by their eyes how the night had gone. She didn't like that aspect of nursing, the way you saw a whole family suffer. In particular, Michele worried about Scott. He looked lost. Some days he was just blank.

If a religious person came into Andrew's room, Michele stayed and sent up a prayer of her own. Sometimes she looked for examples of how God might be reaching down to a patient. In Andrew's case she saw it in all the people who came to see him. She couldn't remember ever seeing so many visitors. She believed that was God's hand. If Andrew survived, she thought he would have plenty of support to keep him on course.

Michele had a standard prayer at bedside. "I'm only human," it went. "Help me do the best I can." Another nurse had an "IV prayer" she would say before putting in a difficult needle. Most nurses were quiet about their particular faith. They supported patients in whatever religion their families had.

Once a week, they had psychosocial rounds in the PICU. Everyone met in a conference room: nurses, techs, even doctors. You could say whatever you wanted and it wouldn't leave the room. A psychiatric nurse-specialist facilitated. A new young doctor might talk about the stress of being up all night. Sometimes people cried. It helped Michele to verbalize things and hear them validated. So much happened in the PICU she believed you really needed to get those feelings out. You certainly couldn't do it during an active resuscitation. Since getting Andrew, Michele had been unable to go to psychosocial rounds; she had to remain at his bedside. She did her best to hold in the day's emotions until her forty-minute commute home. That was when she gave in to it. It wasn't outright sobbing, but it was a release. That way, when she got there, she could give herself back to her own life.

Andrew's wounds continued to be difficult. A few had started to clear on their own, but not most. The toxins caused them to crack and weep. Andrew was covered with dressings that had to be changed regularly. That was one of Kevin Sullivan's jobs. He was thirty-five and had been a nurse two years, switching from hotel-restaurant management. Andrew was Kevin's first meningococcemia case. He did the dressing changes with another nurse.

First they removed the outer Ace wrap, then the four-by-four dressings underneath. Most had become adhered, so they squirted each pad with sterile water before trying to peel it off. Once a wound was uncovered Kevin scrubbed it with a brush, removing dead tissue. Kevin never knew how far down the bad wounds would reach. One on Andrew's upper left arm was necrotic to the bone. It was hard to look at. The bad tissue on his hands reached to the tendons. Orthopedic surgeons were called in to assess permanent damage.

Andrew became agitated during the scrubbing. He would move an arm or leg, or twist his head back and forth. Occasionally he opened his eyes in a shocked way. Kevin at times saw tears. Sometimes they gave Andrew more morphine or Ativan. The room temperature was kept in the mid-eighties to help Andrew maintain circulation. To Kevin, it felt like 100 degrees. He was dripping sweat beneath his gown. The whole process took an hour. They had to do it three or four times a day.

On some shifts, Kevin sat by Andrew's bedside with a calculator, monitoring fluids. He had to track every cc Andrew was getting. Some medications, such as dopamine, had to be counted to the microgram. Kevin watched as Andrew's blood was dialyzed, water filtering out a drop at a time into a collection bag. Occasionally Kevin poured the bag into a measuring beaker so he could compute the amount.

At the end of each hour he added everything up, making sure that the fluid they took off him was just ahead of what they put in. Their goal was to drain 10 cc's per hour, 240 cc's a day, roughly 8 ounces. If they got too far ahead of that, Andrew's blood pressure would drop. If they got behind, fluid would build against his lungs and other organs. Kevin found the work both dull and tense at the same time.

Occasionally it struck Kevin as surprising that Andrew was hanging on at all. This kind of septic shock was often fatal. Kevin wondered if all the praying around Andrew had anything to do with it. Although Kevin had fallen away from the church, it got him thinking again about the role of belief.

Kevin had yet to see Andrew conscious, but he felt he had come to know him anyway. For example, Andrew was hard to sedate, and that told Kevin something about his personality. They gave normal doses of sedation and he'd still be moving, pulling things, thrashing his head. Every so often Andrew got so disruptive Kevin worried he might dislodge his breathing tube. When that happened, Kevin had to hold him by the forehead and ask for someone to please get him some Ativan.

Kevin wrote some of that off to Andrew having built up a tolerance to sedatives, but it was more than that. It fit with the way Rebecca described her son; she said he was a handful. Kevin smiled about it sometimes. Even in a coma Andrew was uncooperative. He didn't want to lie helpless in bed; he wanted to pull things out and be up and running again. It told Kevin that Andrew's personality was still in there somewhere.

Karen Zelano was an ICU nurse who happened to be a family friend. Karen's son had been on the same Little League team as Andrew; her husband and Scott had coached it together. Karen had asked not to be assigned to Andrew, feeling it would be too difficult. She knew him as a spirited kid and was not surprised it showed even as he lay in a coma. But she thought there was more going on than just a high energy level. The thrashing, she believed, was an act of will. It was Andrew's way of battling the disease. Karen believed nurses could tell such things, even with tiny babies. Some just lay there, while others wriggled and bit the ventilator. It became clear which children were fighting hardest to get better.

At shift's end, Kevin reported off to the next team. "Pupils are two and a half millimeters, equal and reactive," he said, indicating that Andrew was neurologically sound. Then a vent rundown: "SIMV mode, rate of 20, ten of pressure support, five of PEEP, title volume of 300." The tube was 4.0, taped at 13 at the lip.

Andrew's heart rate held around 110, and his A-line pressure was 110 over 60, cuff pressure correlating at 112 over 58. Dopamine was at 5 mikes per kilo per minute, epi at .3 mikes. Kevin was unable to palpate any pedal pulses; they needed to be Dopplered instead. Lower extremities were cool to mid-calf. There were no positive cultures, but Andrew remained on antibiotics prophylactically. Abdomen was soft, nondistended, no bowel sounds. Urine output one cc the past twenty-four hours, basically nothing. Andrew remained on 5 percent dextrose solution and half-normal saline for maintenance, 40 cc's per hour. He had a left radial art line and a triple lumen left IJ-three port into his jugular. All the drips were running into his distal port. Kevin went over central venous pressure, then moved on to Andrew's wounds, pointing out where dressings were adhering to skin. Finally, psychosocial issues. Mom and Dad were doing their best. They had their ups and downs.

On July 15, Muhammad Ali visited the PICU. He came into Andrew's room. Despite Ali's Parkinson's disease and being gowned up, Scott felt he had a powerful presence.

Ali asked Scott something. Scott didn't catch it.

"Please?"

Ali asked it again.

Scott still didn't understand. He wasn't sure what to say. He didn't want to be rude about it; this was the heavyweight champion of the world.

On the third try he got it.

"He's six years old," Scott said.

Ali asked what was wrong.

The Batesons did their best to explain.

After he left, Scott sat by Andrew and wondered if the visit might make a difference. He knew some might consider it silly, but mightn't there be healing power in a legend's aura? Mightn't there be, well, some vibration or something that would reach Andrew's subconscious? If you believed in prayer, was it any crazier to believe that a great man's spirit might bring something as well? The possibility gave Scott one more thing to hold on to. He didn't say anything about it, though. He thought people would consider him a bit over the edge.

Andrew often arched his head so far to the right that only one ear, his left, was out of the pillow. He looked almost uncomfortable. Rebecca tried to prop his head straight, but he'd twist right back to that position. Even the nurses had no idea what he was doing. Then they discovered that his right ear was blocked and needed to be cleaned. It convinced Rebecca that he had been turning his head so he could hear from the better ear. That was one more thing that made her wonder about comas.

Mrs. Pinksaw, the kindergarten teacher, finished reading to Andrew. She set down her book. She had faith in God, but couldn't help but wonder why He would let this happen. Then she began thinking about a program they had in kindergarten. It was called Child of the Week. It was centered on a poem titled "I'm Someone Special." Mrs. Pinksaw had borrowed it from a record called *God Made Me Special.* She'd had to take the "God" out because it was public school, but after adapting it she thought the message was still there. It went like this:

I'm someone special, I'm the only one of my kind.

I have a body, and a bright healthy mind,

I have a special purpose that I'm going to find,
I'm someone special, I'm the only one of my kind.

They kept the poem in the middle of the bulletin board. When it was his or her week, each child got to select pictures to put around it. Then Mrs. Pinksaw and the class recited the poem together. The idea was to let the children know how unique they were. Now she remembered the original version of the poem, and thought: *God has a purpose for Andrew.* She believed at that point that he would survive this.

Typically, Father Ken brought Holy Communion in the afternoon. He had come to look forward to seeing Andrew, which was unusual, given his reluctance about hospital visits. This was different. Something was happening around this child. Jesus, Father Ken believed, had reached into the pediatric intensive care unit. Some, Father Ken knew, might feel that he looked too hard for the presence of Christ, but that was his job—and his belief, too. The whole reality of faith, to Father Ken, was to read worldly events beyond the physical to another present dimension.

He saw this around Andrew. He saw God's hand in the way a physician as gifted as Dr. Kleinman had been there for him. He saw it in the ICU staff; despite the relentlessness of this disease, they did not flag. When people under stress displayed such generosity of spirit, that was God's presence—at least to Father Ken it was.

He saw it in Scott and Rebecca too. Sometimes they were in that room twenty, twenty-two hours a day. They may have had their low moments, but they never pushed away. Where did they find the stamina for that, if not through God's grace?

Lynn Cavaliero and Suzanne Kiniry looked into Andrew's room from the nurses' station. Rebecca was at his bedside, along with a priest. It had been two weeks, and there were more folks here now than at the start. Although they were medical professionals, Lynn and Suzanne believed there was such a thing as a healing force. It was hard for them to define, except to say it was different from religion. It was like a mind-body connection. When so many people gathered around a child, telling him he would survive, coma or not, those messages got through. Lynn and Suzanne had seen this before, but never with such intensity. Andrew just lay there. He did not move. The ventilator continued to breathe for him.

Chapter 7

"If your son makes it through the night . . ."

Rebecca stood outside the room where the bone scan was to take place. She watched as they positioned Andrew under the gamma camera. Scott was beside him. The procedure would determine whether Andrew's legs could be saved. Bones that remained healthy would appear white on the machine's computer monitor, while those cut off from circulation would not appear at all. This, Scott and Rebecca understood, would tell the tale.

It was the first time Andrew had been wheeled from the PICU since he arrived fourteen days before. It took a team of eight people an hour and a half to get him ready. His respirator had to come along, as did three IV poles on wheels. Dr. Mindy Morin remained in the unit while her team slowly rolled Andrew down connecting corridors to nuclear medicine.

She was the attending this week, having taken over from Monica Kleinman. It would be up to Dr. Morin to give the Batesons the results. She was not optimistic. A few days before, she had sat down with Scott and Rebecca. "I have to tell you," she said, "the doctors are thinking about Andrew's legs." Scott knew things didn't look so great. When Dr. Charles D'Amato, the orthopedic surgeon, came into the picture, it was a sign. What else would they need him for?

Dr. Morin guessed that Andrew was spiking fevers, in part, because of his legs. She suspected that pseudomonas was growing there, and she worried about *E. coli* and klebsiella. Andrew was getting preemptive antibiotics against such infections, but those could only do so much. Scott understood the situation to be something like gangrene. The scan would make things clear. It was like an X ray, and would determine whether blood flow had stopped. If so, amputation would be the only option. To avoid it would further endanger Andrew's life.

Lisa Tetreault, 29, was the nuclear medicine department's senior technologist. She went into the hot lab and selected a radiopharmaceutical to be injected into Andrew's bloodstream. She drew the appropriate dose of millicuries into a syringe surrounded by a lead shield. In most patients it was injected into the arm and within seconds diffused through the circulatory system. Andrew had plenty of intravenous lines, so she used one of those. The hope was that the radioactive liquid would move down his leg, demonstrating circulation, and eventually light up the bone itself.

Someone mentioned to Rebecca that Lisa Tetreault's son had also had bacterial meningitis. Rebecca asked her what had happened. Her eight-month-old, Alex, had gone into the hospital the previous June. He'd remained there six weeks. The disease caused Alex to have two strokes and several brain surgeries. It left him with a permanent shunt from hydrocephalus. He was still undergoing therapy, and faced developmental deficits.

Lisa decided not to give Rebecca all those details. She did show her a picture of Alex, who looked well. The two talked about the ordeal of a long hospital stay.

"You just take it one day at a time," said Lisa. "One hour at a time."

"Sometimes a minute at a time," said Rebecca.

Rebecca seemed resigned to a bad test result. "He just loved to ride his bike," she said to Lisa Tetreault. "How am I going to tell him that he'll never ride his bike again?"

"You tell him he will," said Lisa. She wasn't sure what else to say.

The gamma camera began to take sequential pictures. Rebecca watched through a window as a whitish gray image of Andrew's blood flow came onto a monitor. It faded as the images moved down the legs. Her sister Deb, in nuclear medicine herself, had been allowed to stand by the monitors. When she came out, Rebecca asked: "Is what we're seeing, what we're seeing?"

"Let's wait until the next scan," said Deb, "and we'll have a better idea."

Three hours later, Andrew was brought back for a second scan. By then the injection would have had time to make its way into all living bone. They again began the gamma camera. The results were pretty clear to everyone in nuclear medicine. No one said much.

A year before, after her son's strokes, they had told Lisa Tetreault that if Alex woke up at all, he would likely be severely brain damaged. That had not happened. She believed that one reason were the prayers Alex had received. All that positive energy, Lisa believed, made a difference. As she moved on to her next patient, she said a prayer of her own for Andrew.

Dr. Morin was outside Andrew's room when an orthopedic doctor brought the films to her. She held them to the light. Andrew's leg bones were lit up from his hips to his knees. Below, the image was black.

"There's nothing," the orthopedist finally said.

Morin just stared. The films made it unambiguous. Quietly, she uttered a four-letter word. There was no longer any doubt.

Mindy Morin grew up outside Boston, and went to medical school at the University of Massachusetts. This was her fourth year as a Hasbro intensivist. She asked Scott and Rebecca if they could join her in the small conference lounge. The parents sat on the couch.

"This is not easy for me to do," Dr. Morin said, "but the bone scan shows the blood flow stops about mid-calf." From the knees down, there was no circulation. Both legs, she said, would have to be amputated. Whether it ended up being above the knee or below, they probably would not know until the surgeon completed the operation.

Although Rebecca had prepared herself, it was still a shock. She started to cry. Scott did too. Rebecca regained control and began to ask about details.

After a few moments, Scott asked whether there was anything the doctors could have done to prevent this.

Dr. Morin said there wasn't. They had tried everything in their power.

"Can't they . . . why is it they have to take the legs off?" asked Scott. "His skin still looks like it's red."

Andrew's circulation, said Dr. Morin, had stopped inside the bone. When that happens, everything dies.

"Well . . ." Scott paused. He groped for some other answer. "Why can't they transplant legs? Someone else's legs?" Logically, he knew this was nonsense, but he was grasping for anything.

"Scott," Dr. Morin said, "I wish that could happen, but there isn't anything like that that we could do." She had learned to be patient in such moments. Dr. Morin said how sorry she was. She wished there was more she could offer.

Scott asked when it would be.

They could wait four or five days to see if the borderline area, the knee, improved enough to be saved. But it would be risky to go beyond that. "At this point," said Dr. Morin, "not amputating his legs is going to make things worse. That could introduce all sorts of infection problems. It could jeopardize his life again."

Scott thought: *It's done. This is it.*

Rebecca and Scott walked to the hospital's garden. Once outside, Scott began pacing. To Rebecca he looked as if he could become violent. She had never known Scott to show his temper physically. This was something new.

It was about 5:30 P.M., July 18. The sun was out. It was a beautiful evening. Scott felt furious inside. Two weeks before, Andrew had been fine. Now he was in a coma with a doctor saying his legs had to be cut off. He supposed Andrew's sports life was over. He had loved tossing a baseball around. Before each toss he would look at Scott with that eye, as if to say, "Let's see if you can catch this one." Andrew also liked slam-dunking a basketball into his Little Tikes net. When Scott came home from work Andrew wouldn't say hi—it was always "Watch this, Dad." Then he would run up the driveway and show off his latest slam-dunk. They had bought the basketball stand when he was two. At the time Andrew hadn't understood what it was, so he'd pushed it down lengthwise and ridden it like a horse. That was typical, thought Scott. Andrew came up with the funniest ways to do things. Now all that was done.

Scott continued to pace. He pictured Andrew sitting in a wheelchair watching the other kids play. Pretty soon Andrew would wake up without the two legs he came into the hospital with. How would they tell him? And where would the amputation points end up? Above the knee? Below? The doctors couldn't say. Scott was sick of that. He was sick of not having any answers. How come Andrew's legs died from having meningitis, anyway? The connection didn't seem logical. What kind of disease did such a thing?

He felt anger building as he paced. Why would God do this to a little boy? He believed God had let him down. That's whose fault this was: God's. He could have stopped it, and didn't. Scott looked upward. "How could You let this happen?" he shouted. And then, even louder: "I hate You. I hate You for this."

He shouted so loudly it frightened Rebecca. She had never seen Scott like this. She wondered if the psychiatrists were watching. There was a trash can near Scott with a rounded metal cover. He slammed his fist onto its top. He hit it as hard as he could. He didn't know why it didn't dent. If his hand was in pain, he didn't notice. Then Scott walked to the swing set and kicked one of the swings. He kept pacing. Everything inside him was tight. He had to walk it off, get the anger out. There was so much of it. He hit the swing again.

"Scott," Rebecca said. "You're scaring me."

Scott didn't answer. He hit the poles holding up the swing set. Then he began to cry.

Rebecca sat with her thoughts. She, too, flashed forward and pictured Andrew in a wheelchair. That would break his heart. She wondered how she would tell him. She was also angry at God. She had always thanked Him for what He had given her, asking in return only to keep what she had. Now He had let her down.

Scott felt overcome again by anger. He swore at God for doing this to a helpless little boy. Scott knew Rebecca wanted him to calm down, but he couldn't. His son was losing his legs. A father would have to be dead inside not to care. He would have to be cold. There was so much fury it left Scott shaking. It was like he had to open a valve to let it out, but didn't know how. At the same time he knew Rebecca had been hit with the same bomb, and she didn't need any more. So he walked away from her.

The family gave Scott and Rebecca a half hour, then began to make their way to the garden. For a while no one said much. Scott ended up near Steve Powers, his brother-in-law. "Steve," said Scott, "how's he ever going to skate and do all those things he's supposed to do? He's never going to be able to play hockey."

Steve's was the hockey family. Even Steve's daughter played. He suspected that was why Scott brought it up. He didn't know what to say in response. It wasn't a time for fake optimism.

"Scott," he finally said, "most of us get up in the morning and put our shoes on. Andrew will get up and put his legs on."

Scott didn't say anything to that.

Soon several dozen people were in the garden, both friends and family. Everyone began to focus on Andrew's knees. Maybe he would be able to keep them. That would be a big plus when it came to prosthetics.

The group remained in the garden until after 10 P.M. Scott was trying to get to the other side of the anger. He knew he needed to focus on what would happen next, but he wasn't able to. He didn't have a clear mind. He felt himself just sinking into this hole. Eventually he went back upstairs.

Rebecca remained in the garden. She was sitting with Deb. "He's on his own," Rebecca said of Scott. "I can't do this anymore." She was shaken by the way Scott had gotten so physical in his anger. He had been so explosive it made Rebecca wonder who he was underneath. She needed a husband who consoled her, not one who lost all control. She told Deb she would probably be keeping more of a distance from him, at least emotionally. She didn't want to put herself in that situation again.

Deb hoped her sister wasn't closing the door completely. If Scott came around, Deb thought, Rebecca would, too. But right now certainly seemed to be a bad time between them.

The next day the Batesons again sat with Dr. Morin. The question of the knees, she said, remained unclear. Were they to do the operation today, they would likely have to amputate above them. But the doctors were okay about putting off surgery in hopes that blood flow there might improve.

What did Dr. Morin think would happen?

Some of the purpura was resolving on Andrew's thighs, the skin there pinking up a bit. If it continued a few inches down, they could perhaps salvage his knees. She couldn't promise it, though. She had her doubts.

Father Ken Letoile arrived for a visit. Things in the room were more somber than usual. The parents told Father Ken it was final, the doctors would have to amputate Andrew's legs. There was an awkward silence. Father Ken prayed for help in knowing what to say, or whether saying nothing was best. It didn't come to him. He stumbled a bit and asked basic questions—when was the operation, that kind of thing. It was a difficult blow to everyone.

Later, Father Ken spoke alone with Rebecca. He asked how she and her husband were doing. Scott, she said, saw this as the beginning of the end. A part of her did, too, but she was moving to a different place, trying to view it as a positive. Andrew's legs weren't alive anymore. They were making him sicker. Once they amputated, perhaps he would get better. The part of him that was causing the fevers would be gone. Maybe, said Rebecca, this would be a turning point.

Father Ken admired Rebecca. It took something extra to see the glass half full at such a time.

Scott kept dwelling on why it had to happen. He could only take so much of "It's going to be fine now." Those kinds of glib assurances made him angry. If people wanted to keep talking that way, Scott was going to take a walk.

Dr. Charles D'Amato, who would be performing the surgery, came daily to check Andrew's legs. He pressed the skin to see if blood flow came back. He took pulses behind the knees. He wanted to give Andrew's body time to see if something might get better. He didn't see many hopeful signs.

Dr. Mindy Morin called in Bill Cioffi for a consult. Cioffi was the head of trauma surgery and a burn specialist. Morin thought he would have an eye for when the risk of infection was getting too high. The two went into Andrew's room. Cioffi was not a big talker. Morin knew him as a talented doctor, and very tough. She respected him, but considered him a hard-ass. Not much seemed to get to him.

When they left the room she was surprised to see that he was having trouble composing himself. Morin had never seen him undone before. He examined burn patients every day, but something about Andrew had reached him.

"Bill," said Dr. Morin, "you have any kids?"

"Yes I do. I have three."

Then he pulled it together and was all business.

"You guys have done a hell of a job," said Dr. Cioffi. "I can't believe this kid made it this far."

They talked a bit about surgery plans. Then Cioffi said, "I don't know how you do this every day, deal with the families. Give them bad news. Walk them through this. I don't know how you do it."

Cioffi was the same doctor who had made Rebecca so angry a week or so earlier.

Both parents, Dr. Morin observed, were on edge. Especially Scott. Counting the days to surgery was tough on them. They had to just sit there and wait.

Scott kept asking the Man upstairs, Why? Had Scott done something wrong? If so, why take it out on Andrew? Why didn't God just take Scott's legs? He had a lot fewer years left on this earth.

Dr. Morin had seen parents react that way before. Hearing that children will lose limbs can hit a mom or dad harder than hearing they might die. You envision your healthy child disabled. That just unhinged Scott.

Scott began to notice a certain look that other parents took on in the pediatric ICU. They would stare but not see things. One mother appeared blank to him. He pictured her as the type who once had sparkling eyes, but there wasn't any sign of that now. Scott wondered whether others looked at him and saw the same thing.

Sometimes Scott thought about the bacteria itself. One moment Andrew was watching fireworks; twelve hours later he was dying. It was as if the disease had no mercy. Rationally, he knew it was just bacteria, but Scott considered it evil. What else would you call such a thing? By the time you got a sign that it was something other than a flu, it was too late. It didn't give you a chance. He wondered if it would have done this had it known Andrew was a child. Maybe it did know. If so, it had no conscience, to attack and destroy a little boy.

Rebecca decided to try a night at the Ronald McDonald House with her daughter, Erin, so the two could be together. Scott had no interest in sleeping there. He would not leave Andrew's room for that long. All he knew was that he needed to be by his son.

The family worried about how Scott was pulling away. If a phone call came in for him, he might just put up a hand. He wasn't up to talking. If he saw the family room full, he might duck past and keep walking. Scott seemed to be out there on his own. No one knew what to do about it.

Scott was the first to admit he wasn't up to chitchat, but he was glad Andrew had that constant flow of support. There was another family there whose son had been in an accident. One morning around two o'clock, Scott began a pot of coffee. He noticed one of the parents asleep on a couch. They'd been there a month and seldom got visitors. The mother seemed like she was just going through the motions. For Andrew's sake, Scott hoped they would not be there so long that people stopped visiting.

The differing reactions of Scott and Rebecca were familiar to Dr. Morin. While mothers sought to nurture a child through illness, fathers showed anger at it. A vigil like this was hard on men; it left them feeling powerless. They tended to beat themselves up, as Scott did. This was his fault, he thought, for not reacting sooner.

Dr. Morin talked about Scott with Monica Kleinman. Both sensed that Scott had a wall around him. During daily meetings he was silent. Mom would ask the questions. Scott appeared lost. A few times he broke down right in front of the team. Mostly he seemed angry. The doctors didn't blame him, but they did worry.

Tracey Guthrie, a hospital psychiatrist, came down daily to check on Scott. She talked to him about those first hours at home.

Scott kept dwelling on the what-ifs. Dr. Guthrie told him he couldn't blame himself; they had brought Andrew in as fast as any reasonable parent would have. Faster, really. Scott nodded.

Guthrie asked if he was eating. How about sleeping? How was he feeling in general?

Not to be rude, but Scott was seldom interested in talking about it. He thought the psychiatrist was nice enough, but it was a waste of words. It didn't matter what anybody said. His son was losing his legs. How did they expect him to feel?

A social worker showed Scott and Rebecca an indentation in the wall. It had been hidden under a poster. It was made by a frustrated father. It was the social worker's way of saying "Reach out if you need us." Scott just looked at the indentation and understood the feeling.

For Rebecca's part, she tried to be up whenever she saw a counselor coming. God forbid they thought she was losing it; they'd put her away.

Karen Zelano, ICU nurse and family friend, was aware of Rebecca's coping strategy. Basically she focused on what needed to be done next. Still, Rebecca had her issues. While Scott pulled inward, Rebecca got obsessive, even overbearing. Every few days, the kidney machine filter needed changing. It was a complex, sterile procedure. Karen was in the room when Rebecca said it was time. The lines appeared clogged.

"Are you going to change it?" Rebecca said to the other nurses.

"Maybe we can get some more out of it the next few hours," one said.

Rebecca snapped at her. "Just change it," she said. "I'll spring for it."

A fellow ICU nurse said to Karen at one point, "I know she's under a lot of pressure, but she's very impatient." Karen just nodded. Rebecca had become all business. There were very few light moments. Karen thought to herself: *That's how she's getting through things, by taking charge.* The staff understood, but sometimes they thought Rebecca came on strong.

Dr. Morin remained concerned about new infection, especially pseudomonas. If that started and spread, Andrew would deteriorate again—crump up, in Morin's words. She knew from Dr. Kleinman that it had happened before. Andrew would stabilize one day and go south the next. He was getting to the point of needing the operation.

At least, thought Rebecca, there had been several days without a medical crisis. That was a positive. Then something happened. Suddenly, Andrew's heart raced and his pressure dropped. One of Rebecca's sisters was in the room, as were two nurses. The four watched the monitors. Andrew's oxygen saturation fell too. What was going wrong? It was so bad they figured the ventilator was malfunctioning. It wasn't. Perhaps a line was clogged then, or kinked, cutting off Andrew's air flow. No, those were fine. Why were Andrew's rates crashing?

Rebecca looked at Andrew and had the sense that he was getting smaller. Several alarms were now beeping. The nurses kept double-checking the respirator. Andrew seemed to get smaller and smaller still. It wasn't Rebecca's imagination. Then everyone saw it. Someone had kicked the air mattress plug out, and it was going down, Andrew sinking into it. They plugged it back in, and soon the bed came back up. As it did, a bit more slowly, Andrew's rates restabilized. You could almost hear the nurses exhale.

Still, it was an unnerving sign. Andrew was so fragile that merely changing his positional support caused him to deteriorate.

Rebecca thought: *He's not really living on his own.* It wasn't just the respirator keeping him alive, even the heated air mattress was. She wondered how long Andrew was going to be in bed, hooked up to machines. She worried it might be like this for a long time.

. . .

131

Not long after, they lost the pulse in Andrew's left wrist. On both hands, his fingers had grown darker. Scott thought: *My God, this can't all be amputated.* He began again to bargain with God. Don't let his hands go, too, he prayed. Who, later in life, would button Andrew's shirts? Put on his shoes? What about typing and driving? Or holding hands with girlfriends? That warm touch to somebody else—that wouldn't be there. How would he brush his teeth and shave? If You have to take something, he prayed, take a foot. But save his hands. Then he grew angry about having to negotiate such trade-offs.

The family had gathered beneath the arbor in the garden. Father Joe was with them. Everyone was feeling down. Early on, it had helped to hear from the priests about faith, but that struck some now as a cliché. Deb told Father Joe she was tired of hearing that bad things happen to good people. Her husband, Steve, was tired of it too. Steve had been questioning God for thirty years. He had long wondered where God was when tragedies happened to children; he said as much to Father Joe. The merciful God he'd been taught about wouldn't do this to a little boy. It made Steve angry. Why was Andrew made sick this way? It was a fair question, wasn't it? And as far as priests saying God never gave you more than you could handle, Steve thought that was a crock. Sometimes God did. Look at Rebecca and Scott. They could barely function, to say nothing of Andrew. He was expected to handle this? Losing his legs? His hands?

Others added similar thoughts. Father Joe just listened. Then he called everyone over, including the parents.

"I want you to hold hands," he said.

The family formed a circle.

"And all say together . . ."

At that, Father Joe suggested a four-letter expletive seldom heard from a priest. In unison, they all began to say it, over and over.

It helped with everyone's tension, and even brought a few

smiles. It also told them Father Joe understood. It was his way of saying there often wasn't an explanation. Sometimes, Father Joe thought, it was all right to just say how furious you were that an appalling thing had happened.

Father Joe saw Scott sitting alone outside on the low stone wall near the hospital entrance. He went to join him. The family had encouraged him to reach out to Scott; others had been unable to connect.

"I know how Andrew is and how Rebecca is," said Father Joe. "How's Scott?"

"I'm doing okay."

"I don't believe you."

"It's hard," Scott said. "I don't know what's going to happen." He talked about what a roller-coaster ride this was. Some doctors thought Andrew would lose just his feet, others said the loss would extend above the knee. One doctor thought he might lose a finger, another the whole arm. Or both arms. Scott no longer knew what he could hope for.

He asked Father Joe how things were at the new parish. Father Joe began to answer, but he could see it wasn't registering.

Scott looked up. "I'm sorry, what did you say?"

Father Joe kept talking anyway. Maybe it was good for Scott to have company while his mind worked in its own direction. After a time, some silences began to fall. Father Joe took it as a hint. He tried to respect when people needed their privacy. He stood to leave.

"Do you have to go?" said Scott.

It struck Father Joe as curious; he had thought Scott was done talking. "Haven't you seen enough of me?" Father Joe said. "I've been here three hours. I have a parish to run."

That got a brief smile out of Scott. Father Joe stayed, the two sitting side by side in silence.

Once Scott asked Father Joe why God couldn't stop this. The two were at a picnic table in the hospital garden. If He brought Lazarus back from the dead, said Scott, why was He allowing this to happen to Andrew?

"Scott, I can't answer you on that one."

Scott took that in. He seemed to respect it. Father Joe found an innocence in Scott; he wasn't a judgmental or mean-spirited guy.

Scott asked about prayer. "We pray," he said, "and I don't see anything happening."

That came back to God having a purpose for things, said Father Joe. "Sometimes our prayer is asking for the grace to accept and trust that."

Scott nodded. Still, he wanted to know what they had done to get punished like this. It made him want to scream.

"These things don't happen as a punishment," said Father Joe. A lot of life could not be explained. Then he told Scott about his brother, Russell, who had been killed three years before in a car accident. He left a wife and three children. Russell had been thirty-one. It happened on Thanksgiving Day, 1994, in Maine. Afterward, a sister-in-law told Father Joe she didn't think something like that could happen to Russell because his brother was a priest. "As if being a priest," Father Joe told Scott, "was an insurance policy against anything bad in the family."

The story seemed to hit a chord. Scott asked Father Joe how he dealt with it. "You deal with it each day," said Father Joe. "There were days I didn't want to get out of bed in the morning. There were days I had no patience with people. There were days I've been unhappy with how things turned out in my life. But you need to grow with it," he said. "You can't change it. You can't just invest your energy being angry about it." Scott listened. He said he appreciated Father Joe being so honest.

Father Ken Letoile tried to help Scott too. While in the garden one day they got to talking about God—how angry Scott was at Him. Father Ken said it was normal to feel that way. Besides, he said, anger is a venerable emotion. There was certainly enough of it in the Bible.

"If you open up the Book of Psalms," said Father Ken, "I don't know what the percentage is, but there's a lot of anger at God in those Psalms." God can take it, he told Scott. God understood where the anger was coming from.

Scott asked why God would do this to Andrew? A little boy?

"Jesus didn't cause this disease, Scott," said Father Ken. "He never would have chosen this for your son. He's angry about this too." Illness, he explained, was a contradiction to God's kingdom. That was not where to look for His hand. Rather, it lay in the strength one can feel when things were bleakest. That was the presence of Christ.

Scott didn't say anything. Father Ken could tell he wasn't convinced. So he talked about a doctor as skilled as Monica Kleinman having been there at the right time. He spoke of Jesus working through all these human instrumentalities to bring hope to a situation marked by tragedy.

What about now, Scott asked. Look at what was happening to Andrew's legs.

Father Ken answered: "Jesus sucks it up and says, 'I don't like this either, but the only way we can preserve Andrew's quality of life is amputation. He's still got his brain, his heart, everything else he needs to be human.'"

Scott didn't say much more. Father Ken put his arm around him. He could tell Scott remained far away. After a few moments, Father Ken stood. "I'll see you upstairs."

Father Ken was inclined to be a fixer by nature. It was difficult for him to run into situations where he couldn't be of much help.

Karen Lamberton saw her brother Scottie as lost. He had always prided himself on appearance, but most days now his shirt was untucked and his hair unkempt. He was often in a chair, hunched over, his head down. He seemed to have no spirit. Karen's husband, John, felt it all had sucked the soul right out of him. Several family members said "Scott's gone off." That was how they put it.

Jimmy Bateson, Scott's older brother, worked maintenance at

Amica. He took a chunk of his vacation to spend time with Scott at the hospital. It was a hard few days. Scott frequently broke down. He often said, "I don't know what I'm going to do." Jimmy couldn't remember Scott being depressed, even briefly. He was by nature a cheerful guy. This was something new. None of the family had seen him like this.

Jimmy tried to coax Scott to open up, but he didn't get far. He thought his brother held a lot in, and always had. When he was younger, if he had problems at school—like some kid picking on him—you'd never know. He didn't talk about what was going on inside.

Scott's father, Jim, 72, was visiting in Andrew's room. He noticed Scott wasn't there. He went out of the room to look for him. Way down at the end of the corridor, outside the PICU, was Scott. He was sitting by himself in a chair. Jim walked down and sat next to his son. He asked Scott how he was doing.

"I had so many things planned for him," said Scott. "He was going to play baseball." Scott mentioned other sports.

"Scott," said his dad, "you have to wait and see."

To George, a younger brother, Scott seemed in a kind of disbelief.

"I was going to New Hampshire," he said, "and now a doctor's saying, 'If your son makes it through the night . . .'"

Scott's family saw Rebecca as the stronger one at this time. In his mind, George traced it to the different ways the two came up. If someone broke a glass in the Bateson family, they'd spend a lot of energy regretting that it happened. Rebecca's family, George thought, would just clean it up. The hospital, George thought, brought out those two different mind-sets.

George also observed that while some families had a lot of tragedies, theirs hadn't. Then Scott got a one-two: Their mother had died sixteen months before, in February of 1996, and now this.

Once Scott was sitting at the hospital with his sister Karen. "I wish Mom was here," he said. He believed she would know what to say. Scott, Karen thought, had relied on their mom's comforting, and she wasn't there now. The way Scott's sister-in-law Lori Bateson saw it, mothers had a job, and fathers had a job. This was a time when, even as an adult, you needed your mother. It was hard for Scott not to have one.

Chapter 8

"Andrew needs Your help right now . . ."

Rebecca thought about those TV movies where the husband and wife seemed so together in a crisis. That wasn't Rebecca and Scott. The two were in different worlds. They seldom spent time just with each other, and when they did they barely talked—at least, not the way couples do. Rebecca didn't feel very married. At times, Scott's anger continued to unnerve her. Mostly, he brooded. It was the loneliest Rebecca remembered feeling. It became a physical ache in her chest.

In her view, Scott wasn't someone she could lean on at the moment. Rebecca was the one who had to be strong. She wished she didn't have to play that role. She wanted just to go outside and scream. It was tiring to have to stay levelheaded. She was angry that Scott wasn't a rock to her. That's what she wanted in a husband right now.

It was ironic in a way, since she had married Scott for his sensitivity. She remembered one of their first dates: He drove her to the resort town of Newport, Rhode Island, where they strolled by the ocean, then went back to his car, which Scott had parked by a low wall near some tourist shops. He opened the trunk. Inside there was a picnic lunch. He had put together this whole nice layout— sandwiches, fruit, even chilled wine. It wasn't overly fancy, which Rebecca thought was good; otherwise it would have meant he had done it before with another woman. They sat on the wall and picnicked right there. Rebecca liked that, too. Other guys might not have done this in a public place, but Scott wasn't shy about showing affection.

He had a nice car at the time, a Buick Presidential. Five weeks after they began dating, he decided to sell it. He didn't have tons of money, so it was the only way he could afford a ring. Rebecca was twenty-four, Scott ten years older. It was 1985.

Rebecca didn't have to think twice about saying yes. She knew he was the right one, mostly because of that untypical side of him, the way he didn't constantly talk sports, or act like she didn't matter when he was with male friends.

Although he would later deny it, Rebecca remembers him crying a little at the altar. Scott didn't seem afraid to wear it on his sleeve. That's what she wanted, not the macho man who acted tough no matter what.

But now, in the hospital, that was exactly what she wished Scott would be: a tough guy who would tell her everything would be okay, even if he didn't believe it. She wanted him to make the decisions, handle things. She wanted to be the child, not the adult. Rebecca thought she had lost that partner whose shoulder she could lay her head on.

Their friends couldn't help but notice a distance between them. To Maria Amaral, Scott had pulled away. Perhaps, Maria thought, that's how men were. They had to do their grieving on their own.

"Scott's gone off," was how Rebecca put it.

"This is his moment," replied Maria. "When you have your moment, he'll be the strong one."

Once Rebecca made a joke about it. She said she didn't know how to talk to him anymore, though maybe it was because they were married. Didn't you lose your communication skills at the altar?

Maybe, Maria thought, Scott and Rebecca couldn't be expected to stay connected. They were both giving all they had to Andrew and didn't have anything left for one another.

...

Cindy Day, from across the street, felt for Scott. It broke her heart to see a man so torn up. A few times Scott told her about his fears that Andrew would be wheelchair bound. Maybe, Cindy thought, this was how fathers worked out their grief: they pictured the worst case. Cindy imagined all the athletic things Scott once hoped to share with his son. Now, in Scott's mind, those were out the window. His whole focus was on loss, and it made him withdraw.

Cindy understood Rebecca, too. At a time like this a woman wanted her man to be bulletproof. Cindy certainly would.

She couldn't blame either one. Both parents were too broken to accommodate the other, and resentful at not being understood. Having a sick child would test any marriage, Cindy thought. She hoped the Batesons would get through it.

From their posts at the nurses' station, Suzanne Kiniry and Lynn Cavaliero also saw Scott and Rebecca drift apart. Pediatric intensive care units, the two supervisors knew, destroyed marriages. Both had sat there and watched it happen. Women and men often coped differently, the female needing support, the male needing space, both angry that the other was at such an opposite place. Neither Suzanne nor Lynn had a good feeling about how Scott and Rebecca would end up.

There had been plenty of husbands the nurses found unappealing. Scott was different. Karen Zelano never heard a nasty word about him among the staff. Many men, although withdrawn, still put on a front. Scott let you see through. He would come back from a shower looking refreshed, gown up, and if things had gotten worse his body just sagged. He seemed broken and didn't try to hide it. The nurses felt for him.

Once Scott said to Suzanne Kiniry, "When am I going to be able to do this, walk in here and not cry?"

He seldom shared such thoughts with Rebecca, which Suzanne found typical. It was as if men thought: *She doesn't need to deal with the fact that I can't deal with this.* So around their wives, men turned inward, and the wives felt abandoned.

Karen Zelano knew that Rebecca had an issue with Scott's anger. But Scott wasn't the first such father Karen had seen in the ICU. Once, after getting bad news about his child, she saw a dad put a fist through a hospital wall. They'd had to call security to take him out. He was just a regular middle-class guy.

For weeks people had been pushing Scott and Rebecca to go out to dinner. They resisted until the priests pushed too. Neither was good at saying no to a priest; it was that whole Irish-guilt thing. Rebecca insisted it be someplace close. They settled on a restaurant called Angelo's, a mile away. They went with Manny and Maria Amaral.

As soon as they got in the car Rebecca grew anxious. She hoped it would be over soon. Someone must have talked to Angelo's because they walked right to a table, despite it being a Saturday night. People tried to make conversation, but it made Rebecca uncomfortable to have an enjoyable time while Andrew couldn't. She asked everyone to look at the menu and decide. Scott said little. He wasn't really focusing. The meal came quickly, though it didn't seem so to Rebecca.

Scott grew increasingly uptight. The outing made him think about how hard normal moments like this would now be.

"Guys," Rebecca soon said, "we've got to go." She felt a bit rude, as no one had finished. They motioned for the check, paid it, and left. Scott and Rebecca asked to be dropped off at the hospital door before the Amarals parked. They took the elevator to the intensive care unit, and went back to Andrew's room. When they at last stepped inside, it was almost with a feeling of relief.

Rebecca tried to find a way to be optimistic. She thought about stories of handicapped people who seemed able to do anything, or those like Christopher Reeve who didn't give up. She tried to draw from such folks. Rebecca thought she had to be okay with this in front of Andrew—or at least be able to act like she was. She didn't want him surrounded by some funeral gathering when he woke up. Mentally, she made a point of thinking "when," not "if."

One technique that worked for Rebecca was to pray for Andrew's knees. It gave her a positive goal. If they could not save his legs, at least let them keep his knees. She tried to be realistic that way.

A nurse told the Batesons of a ritual another couple had tried. They had placed a cloth scapular on their child. It had a picture of the Virgin Mary on one side and a prayer on the other. It was the size of a business card and supposedly had healing significance. In the other couple's case, things had turned out well. The nurse didn't want to say it was a miracle or would make a difference with Andrew but sensed it was along the lines the Batesons had been thinking.

Scott asked the two priests if they had such scapulars. They did. Both parents thought the idea was a little out there, but they tried it anyway. After each dressing change, they placed the scapulars on Andrew. They put them on his arms and his legs. Rebecca usually placed them a few inches below his knees. She taped them on to make sure they wouldn't fall off.

Scott had never been overly religious, never wore crosses, so this was different, using the scapulars this way. Then again, he had done something similar with a small statue right after Andrew went into the hospital. A friend had offered to get clothes for the Batesons from their house. Scott asked if she wouldn't mind bringing something else. There was a statue of Jesus holding a heart next to their bedroom bureau. Could she get that too? It was about fifteen inches high and made of painted plaster. It had belonged to Scott's grandmother. She used to pray over it every afternoon, even if Scott was visiting. She kept the statue on a dresser between two dark maroon votive cups. Scott would sit there and listen to her going along the rosary. Every day for her, that had to happen.

Scott was close to his grandmother. You know how with certain people, you get along? That was Scott and his grandmother. She lived near his family in East Providence. Sometimes, as a kid, he used to run to the grocery to do shopping for her. When he got back that statue always caught his eye; it struck him as having some kind of life. It was as if those eyes could see. Scott never prayed before it himself. Well, perhaps once or twice as a kid if there was something he really needed help with. But he wasn't a holy jumper or anything.

Scott was in his late twenties when his grandmother passed away. As they were starting to break up her house Scott told his mother, "Ma, if there's one thing you can get for me, it would be that statue." He thought it would be a nice connection to his grandmother.

At the hospital he put it on a window shelf behind Andrew. It had never been Rebecca's favorite item; it was a little taller than she liked her statues. She found it slightly creepy, with that heart dripping blood. But she knew it meant something to Scott so she didn't say anything. Perhaps, she thought, it might even help. At first the statue stood alone on the window ledge. After a week or so Rebecca thought it looked like E.T. in the closet. That was how many stuffed animals they had gotten.

Scott resisted praying just for Andrew's knees. He felt that would be giving in. He continued asking that Andrew's whole legs be healed. He did so three times a day in the chapel.

"If You hear me," Scott prayed, "Andrew needs Your help right now. He's in a bad way." He asked God to make it so this didn't have to happen. Then he prayed for Andrew's hands. If God had to take something, prayed Scott, please don't let it be those.

He remembered what Father Ken had said about reading the Psalms. Scott hadn't looked at a Bible for years. Now he thumbed through it, the Psalms anyway, and did find some helpful passages.

People tried to buck up the Batesons with success stories about prosthetics. One woman gave them a videocassette. Scott and Rebecca put it aside; they weren't ready to see it. They didn't want to visualize what that would look like. To both it felt like a betrayal of Andrew to plan for him without legs before it actually happened. Cindy Day understood. Everyone wanted to harp on the "woulds"—that even without legs, Andrew would walk again, would bike again, would be normal again. It was well meaning, but Cindy thought it too early for that.

Andrew's operation was a few days away. Scott still hoped God would stop it. He got the idea to go to St. Francis Chapel in downtown Providence. Maybe praying at a church would be more effective. Scott remembered St. Francis from an earlier visit. It had religious statues around the walls representing different saints. You lit a candle in front of each and said a prayer. People had attached notes saying, for example, that St. Peter had helped with these two requests, and on like that. Scott knew you didn't have to pray in front of a statue for God to hear you, but maybe this would give it some extra punch.

Scott approached a friend of theirs who had stopped for a visit. If it wasn't too much trouble, could she take him to St. Francis? He got in her van. It was Scott's second trip off the property, and the first in daytime. It felt funny driving into the city. Seeing the busy downtown pace was jarring; people rushed through their business as if nothing had happened.

There were only a few people inside St. Francis. He walked to one of the statues. It seemed odd talking to a plaster figure, but at this point Scott was open to anything. Maybe there was a chance it would let the saints know what he was asking for.

"God," he prayed, "please come in and take Andrew and heal him, You know, come and touch him. Make his legs heal, and his hands. And please let him survive."

He went to the next statue, lit the candle, and made a similar prayer. He did so in front of most of them. When Scott was done he asked an attendant if there was a priest he could speak to. After a few minutes an older gentleman came out. He had on a robe. He must have been a friar, though, to be honest, Scott wasn't sure what they called them.

"How can I help you?"

Scott explained about Andrew. As he talked the friar escorted him past the statues to a back room. It was just the two of them. It sure would be good, thought Scott, to have the assistance of a man of this level. "The reason I came," said Scott, "was to ask for some kind of help; if, somehow, you could maybe pray for Andrew at a Mass." The priest said he would do so. Then he told Scott to go into the chapel again, to the back, where there was a chalice. He told Scott to pray before it, touch it, then touch Andrew with that hand and ask that God heal him.

Back at the hospital, Scott touched Andrew's legs just as the friar had asked.

The Batesons got to know other PICU families. One baby boy had been born without an esophagus. He was already a patient when Andrew arrived. He had been intubated at the time, and remained so. Now the doctors planned to remove the breathing tube the next day. "That's good," Scott told the mom and dad. "Maybe you guys will get out of here real soon." That was a common theme among PICU families, the hope of leaving. As the procedure was about to begin, Scott and Rebecca stood beside the little boy's parents, who had been advised to wait outside the room. After a while the doctor came out to say he was sorry, but the baby had not breathed on his own. They'd had to put the tube back in. The mother broke down at the news. Rebecca held her. It was a big disappointment. Scott understood about having hope and then getting knocked backward.

Linda Snelling was the third intensivist. She viewed her week's purpose as seeing Andrew through surgery. She was approaching her tenth year in this work. To her, it had a reward that you found less often in some adult ICUs. You could take patients who looked like they might die, and if you gave them good care they could have a normal life. Andrew was not such a child. Even if they could save him he would not leave the way he came in. It was frequently like that with meningococcemia. Dr. Snelling saw it as a particularly unfair disease.

A few times Snelling heard staffers tell the Batesons they were lucky; many kids died from this, and there was a chance Andrew would lose only his legs. She considered such comments well intentioned but cruel. It told Scott and Rebecca that they weren't entitled to grieve. Snelling chose to give them a different message. She told the parents there was nothing lucky about this situation. It was a horrendous thing. It didn't mean Andrew's life was over, but things would not be as they were. Some thought she was too direct, but Snelling believed a doctor should acknowledge despair.

Dr. Snelling sat down with the parents in the consultation room. Some specialists were there too. It was 10 A.M., right after rounds. She told the Batesons that Andrew was assisting the ventilator, a good sign. They wanted to try extubating him to see if he could breathe on his own. This surprised Rebecca. There was a question about that? She assumed Andrew was different from the baby who didn't have an esophagus; all they had to do was lighten his coma and pull the tube, and he'd be fine.

Rebecca asked: Why now, before surgery?

Because the longer he was on the respirator, the more likely he would develop trauma to his trachea, which could leave it permanently narrowed.

What if he could not breathe well enough without the machine?

They would give him some time to declare himself. If he remained distressed, they would reintubate him.

The doctors advised that the parents not be in the room. Rebecca did not argue.

It was a full house: Dr. Snelling, several residents, and a respiratory therapist. They closed both the door and the window blinds. About five minutes later, Snelling came out. She was sorry, but they'd had to reintubate. As soon as the tube was removed, Andrew's throat had swollen closed. It shook Rebecca. That was one more thing to worry about.

Several days later they attempted it again. This time they left the blinds open.

"I can't look," said Rebecca. She turned her back to the room. Still, she wanted to know.

Karen Zelano agreed to help her through it.

"They're taking out the tube," said Karen. "They're suctioning. . . . They're listening with their stethoscopes. . . . They're standing over the bed watching him . . . looking at the monitors . . . looking at him."

The first time Andrew failed at this, he declared himself right away. It was slower this time.

"They're putting an oxygen mask on him. . . ."

Then they called it. It wasn't working. They had to reintubate yet again. There was some concern that Andrew's throat might be affected by meningococcal lesions. Rebecca felt mostly numb.

With the operation approaching, Father Ken proposed a healing Mass at St. Pius, the Batesons' church in Providence. They would pray for Andrew's health, he said, and for his knees. He was a bit surprised when Scott and Rebecca said they would leave the hospital to attend. The Mass took place Sunday, July 20. It began at 10 A.M. The church was full.

Father Ken wore the green robes appropriate from June through Thanksgiving. He said they had gathered to call upon Jesus to be present to Andrew, who would be operated upon Tuesday.

Scott and Rebecca sat in the second pew. In front of the altar there was a cross with the figure of Jesus during the crucifixion. Scott decided to picture the figure as God Himself and direct his prayers right there. He prayed not just for Andrew's knees, but that his whole legs be healed.

The gospel that day was John, Chapter 6. The Scripture was about Jesus working through a young boy to feed a multitude, which struck Father Ken as a sign. Following the readings, Father Ken preached a homily. Then there was a reflection from the Batesons. Rebecca said they had witnessed three miracles: that Andrew was alive, and so far had both his mind and his hands. "For this," she said, "we are eternally grateful to God."

To hear gratitude at such a moment struck Father Ken as a deep statement of faith. He wept as he listened.

About 1,000 people had come for the Mass. To Scott, it felt strong, everyone praying together. There was a lot of power in that church. Father Ken hoped it told the family that Christ was at their side. The energy that was in the church spilled outside, where refreshments were set up on the front lawn. It was a beautiful summer day. Father Ken sensed a greater sense of community among parishioners than he had seen in his ten years at St. Pius. This little boy had brought Christ's love here in a way he had never felt so keenly.

The orthopedic surgeon, Charles D'Amato, visited often as the operation date approached. At one point he mentioned Andrew's hands. The index finger on his right hand was quite black, at least the last digit. He suggested that when the amputations were done, they might want to look at a part of that finger at the same time.

Scott and Rebecca asked if it might not improve.

There was a theoretical chance, said D'Amato. So yes, they would leave it as it was and see what it did on its own. But he wanted to be honest with them.

What did D'Amato think about Andrew's other fingers? And hands?

There may be no need to amputate, he said, but he was pessimistic about function. He worried that Andrew would not gain back much use of the hands. There had been damage right down to the tendons. Often, that was permanent. He didn't want Scott and Rebecca to get their hopes up.

Dr. Snelling went over the operation with the parents. As terrible as this was, said Snelling, it was part of getting Andrew better.

Rebecca asked how well he would be able to function as an amputee.

"He's a kid," said Snelling. "If you don't get in his way, he can do anything."

Would there be a difference if they couldn't save his knees? Dr. Snelling didn't want to lie to them. Saving his knees would make a big difference.

Andrew had six IV lines, and, more than ever, looked like a burn patient. Most of his body was still covered with bandaging. They continued to scrub off the bad skin twice a day. After they rebandaged him, Scott and Rebecca put the cloth scapulars back on. They placed them about four inches below Andrew's knees.

Chapter 9

"It's in God's hands . . ."

The night before the operation, July 21, Scott and Rebecca were in Andrew's room when Dr. D'Amato came in. It was around eleven o'clock. He had forms he needed signed. The three walked to the nurses' station. Rebecca was taken aback by one reference. It said the amputations would probably be above the knee on both legs. That was the plan? She thought it was being left open. Didn't the bone scan put the blood flow at the knee?

Dr. D'Amato said it was very close.

"You have to save his knees," Rebecca said.

"I want the best for Andrew," Dr. D'Amato said. "We're going to save every bit we can." But in these types of situations, he said, it's usually above the knee.

Scott felt knocked to the ground. Lately, to brace himself, he had tried to focus on all the extra activities Andrew would be able to do with knees. *Here we go again*, he thought.

Dr. D'Amato said it wasn't something he could control. If the bone was necrotic, it would have to go. He would not be able to tell where that was until he got in. It was late, and Dr. D'Amato seemed tired. He told Rebecca he had just studied his schedule for the next day and, to be honest, wasn't sure he would be able to do the operation. A lot of things had come up, and it would be tough to squeeze it in.

"I don't care if it's ten o'clock at night," said Rebecca. "You can't do this to me another day."

He seemed surprised at the pressure.

"Do you want me to do this exhausted?" he asked.

"You're a doctor."

He nodded. He promised to look at his schedule again and try to do the operation midday.

The papers lay there in front of the Batesons.

"I can't do this," said Scott. He didn't mean he refused permission; he just didn't have the heart to say officially, "Amputate my son's legs."

Rebecca took the pen. She asked if D'Amato would add a phrase saying he'd amputate above the knee only as a last option. D'Amato did so. But he couldn't be optimistic.

Quickly, Rebecca signed.

Scott thought he should have stepped up to that job. He didn't want to be weak about this, but maybe he was, he admitted to himself.

The parents spent the night in the room with Andrew. Earlier, Dr. D'Amato had told them of a boy they thought would lose only toes but ended up losing a leg above the knee. That kind of petrified Rebecca, that there could be that much of a discrepancy.

Scott woke up before light at Andrew's bedside. They started getting him ready around 10 A.M. It was a long process. Scott paced. The skin on Andrew's legs looked bad. Scott had hoped for some kind of miracle. He had prayed really hard for that. He had asked and asked, but it hadn't happened. For some reason, he no longer felt angry about it.

As the nurses converted the equipment to portability, Scott thought about Andrew playing baseball. They had just finished their first year of Little League. He pictured Andrew running out a single. Andrew had also done soccer the previous fall. Scott pictured that, too—Andrew sprinting on a soccer field—but then that image grayed out.

Monica Kleinman came into the unit. She was not on service but had kept up with Andrew daily. Now she wanted to talk to the parents.

"Guys," Dr. Kleinman said, "I told you before that I'd tell you when I thought Andrew was out of danger and will live. Well, I'm looking you in the eye now, and telling you he will survive."

Kleinman wasn't guaranteeing anything, since a bolt of lightning could strike anyone at any moment. But as far as dying from the infection, he was getting out of that danger zone.

It was odd, thought Rebecca, to get such news and not be able to celebrate because of what was about to happen.

The operating room was down the corridor from the pediatric ICU. They began to move Andrew at about 2 P.M. Scott held on to the rolling gurney and wouldn't let go. Mike Day was nearby, and so was Father Ken. All the two men could say was "Come on, Scott." He kept moving with the gurney, through two sets of doors. Mike and Father Ken tried to stop him from going through the final set. That was for medical personnel only. It was an emotional moment. Scott was holding on and just sobbing.

"Come on, Scott," they said again. Mike told him there was nothing they could do at this point. It was in the doctor's hands.

"It's in God's hands," said Father Ken.

The nurses wheeled Andrew's bed through the final set of doors.

From time to time in her life, Rebecca had heard people talk about that feeling where your legs go weak, but she had never experienced it. Now she did. She started to collapse. Scott caught her. The doors closed. Neither parent said anything.

Having been Andrew's nurse from the start, Michele Rozenberg escorted him in. The journey was a symbolic one. Everybody knew

Andrew was going to be different after this. You couldn't pretend it wasn't happening. The operating room doors closed after him. Michele didn't want anyone to see her reaction. She didn't mind patients knowing she was human, but thought it was inappropriate to cry openly; that would put a burden on the family to comfort her. She kept it together until Scott and Rebecca began to walk away. Then Michele ducked into an area where OR patients changed clothes. She closed the door of a cubicle and sat there alone for a few minutes. Then she collected herself and went back to work.

Dr. Mindy Morin remained in the ICU. She had spoken to Charlie D'Amato as they were wheeling Andrew out of the unit. D'Amato said he did not know whether he would have to take the knees or not. Dr. Morin shared this with some of her colleagues. As she went about her work, Morin kept thinking, *Man, what is going to happen in there?*

Everyone went into the surgical waiting room. It was mostly family, but Mike Day from across the street and Father Ken were there too. Rebecca sat by a small bulletin board. There was a flyer on it about child safety—swimming, bicycling, and such. She read it in English, then tried to read it in Spanish. Nearby there was a painting of an old carousel. There was another of a boardwalk in Newport in the 1920s, with colorful umbrellas along the beach. A third time, and then a fourth, Rebecca reread the flyer on the bulletin board.

Scott got up to walk to the garden. Mike Day went with him. Mike tried to get Scott's mind off it, talking about his last shift at the fire department. Scott didn't say much. Mike tried telling him that Andrew was young and would adjust. It didn't really work. Scott was too upset. A few times the two men sort of cried together. Mike kept that to himself.

Scott wondered what this would do to Andrew mentally. Would he become a sad child? Andrew was always flying out the door, racing around with his friends. How could he do that anymore? The family had gone skiing the previous winter. Andrew had had one chance at it, and that was that. Scott kept checking the time. Earlier, the hours before surgery had flown by. Now each minute seemed to crawl.

Father Ken sat next to Rebecca in the waiting room. Things were quiet. Occasionally someone left for coffee, then returned. No one really talked. This wasn't a good time for reassurances. They were all aware that it could go either way. Every forty-five minutes or so, a nurse came out to say things were moving along, though there was nothing yet to report. Eventually most folks ended up outside the hospital's entrance, just for air.

Scott was still in the garden. How, he wondered, would they tell Andrew? He could not imagine how a parent explains such a thing to a child.

Around 4 P.M., Dr. D'Amato sent a nurse out to report to the family. Soon she found the group at the hospital's entrance. Everyone but Scott was there. The nurse said they had finished one of Andrew's legs. They had been able to save the knee. They had also saved four inches below the knee. There was a cheer, as if a football team had scored a touchdown. A number of people held hands, including Father Ken, and quietly gave thanks. Mike Day went to tell Scott.

Then things became strained again. It was another hour before the nurse came back out. She announced that they had saved the second knee as well, and four inches below it. Andrew needed that much for prosthetics, and now he had it. There was another cheer. Father Ken started to weep. Then he looked up. "I knew it, God," he said. "I knew it." The nurse said it would be another hour or two before Andrew was sutured and in recovery.

Father Ken proposed a Mass of thanksgiving. They gathered in the chapel. Father Ken did not doubt that the doctors could explain the saving of Andrew's knees medically, but he looked at it through the eyes of faith, and saw this as a sign of Christ's hand.

To Rebecca, everything felt lighter. It was as though she could breathe again.

After the Mass, people went back to the garden and new visitors soon showed up, including Father Joe Escobar. Mike Day disappeared, then returned with twenty steak sandwiches from the popular Twin Oaks restaurant. He brought french fries and onion rings too. It was the best dinner Scott remembered having. It was the only meal since the beginning that he really tasted. It was the family's eighteenth day in the hospital.

Father Joe realized it was the first time he had heard laughing among the family. Even Scott smiled once or twice. The two strolled off together.

"You doing all right?"

"I'm afraid to be too happy," said Scott.

"Well, you got good news today. You need to celebrate that. That's not to say there won't be bumps in the road, but this is good."

"Yeah," Scott said, "you're right." Scott had prayed for more, but he thought that saving Andrew's knees was possibly a miracle of sorts.

Father Ken lingered later than usual. He was a Dominican friar, having graduated from the Dominican House of Studies in Washington, D.C. He thought back to when he first experienced a closeness to God as an altar boy. It was what drew him to this work, and he felt it again now.

Rebecca and Scott went up to see Andrew, who had been settled back in the room. The nurses said he was doing well, but would be in a deeper coma due to the extra anesthesia for surgery. Dr. D'Amato came by. He looked wiped out. The three went to the hallway to talk. It was about 9 P.M.

D'Amato was pleased with the way the operation had gone, but he had a concern. There wasn't a whole lot of bone below the knee. Just *enough*. However, he had cut at the border of bad tissue, which was a risk. If an infection developed, that would change things. He had loaded the ends of Andrew's legs with antibiotic beads. Andrew was due back in the OR for a surgical exam in three days. D'Amato would know then if he needed to take more.

To Scott, it was like they'd had this one hour to exhale and now needed to hold their breath again. Still, Scott knew this would help make Andrew well. He tried to think about that as he headed back to the garden.

Father Joe lingered late. Before he left, he told Scott he was going upstairs to see Andrew. He wanted to carry the feeling into the room. Father Joe was the lone visitor. He gowned up and pulled a stool to the side of the bed. It was a quiet time medically.

"Andrew, it's Father Joe. You had a big day today. You had your surgery. Everything went well."

Father Joe believed that on some level Andrew was aware of him. He remembered sitting with another boy in a coma, Brian Feeney. In that case Father Joe had held the boy's feet and told him to push. Brian did. That told Father Joe that Brian was still in there somewhere.

Andrew's hands were resting on his stomach. Father Joe took one of them in his own hand. "I'm going to say a prayer with you," he told Andrew. "You just relax." He made the sign of the cross, closed his eyes, and prayed the rosary in thanks: "In the name of the Father, the Son, and the Holy Spirit . . ."

To himself, Father Joe prayed the apostle's creed: "I believe in God the Father almighty, the maker of heaven and earth. I believe in Jesus Christ, His only son. . . ." One by one, he went through each rosary bead, giving thanks. "Hail Mary, full of grace . . ."

The session took fifteen minutes. After finishing, Father Joe sat there thinking about what Andrew's life would be like. Then an image came to him. He pictured Andrew as a young man on his wedding day, standing in his tuxedo at the foot of the aisle, waiting for his bride. It was a very clear image: Andrew Bateson as a groom.

Father Joe again made the sign of the cross, and headed home.

. . .

That night Rebecca decided to sleep in the Ronald McDonald House for the first time. Dr. Kleinman's assurance made her feel she could. She got there about midnight. It was quite a nice place. The room was small but had a homey feel. She lay down and thought about how she no longer had to pray for Andrew's legs. She did pray a little for his knees, though, given Dr. D'Amato's concern.

The next morning Rebecca noticed other folks in the courtyard. She watched them talking among themselves, and could just tell. Apparently, they were there to see things through to the end. It made her think that in one sense, she did not have it so bad.

Kevin Sullivan was in Andrew's room the next day on his regular nursing shift. It struck him that when they amputated, it was just below where Scott and Rebecca had consistently placed the scapulars. He pointed this out to his colleague, Claire Piette. "What do you think?" he asked.

"I don't know," Claire said. "I don't know if that was a coincidence."

They agreed it probably was. It had to be.

Over the next days, Andrew's fever began to subside. His white count improved, too. Slowly, he seemed to be stabilizing. It made Scott realize how important the operation had been.

Dr. D'Amato's post-surgical check would be an important test. If they had cut too low, there would be chronic infection problems. That would require more amputation and would change things. For below-knee prostheses to work, Andrew needed to keep most of what he had. There was little margin for more loss.

For Scott, the three-day wait went slowly. All the old fears came back. His whole focus was that surgical check.

They had scheduled it for 2 P.M., but some emergencies delayed Dr. D'Amato. Scott grew anxious. An hour went by, then two, and three. Scott must have paced the corridor a thousand times. The dinner hour passed, and then it got dark. By now Scott was drained. He was walking the corridor when some friends, a couple, came up to him. The husband said, "Scott, you have to be strong."

That finally did it.

"What the hell do you think I've been?" Scott said. He was almost yelling. "I've been here since July Fourth. My son's lost two legs, I've been waiting eight hours for the OR, and you're telling me to be strong? If that's what you got to say to me, don't say anything."

He had to walk away then. That really sent him. It just wasn't the right thing to tell him at all.

D'Amato was finally ready at 10:30 P.M. He followed Andrew into an operating room. It was midnight when he came out. He had to take a bit off the bone of one leg, debride a little dead tissue, but it was minimal. Generally things looked fine, he said. Andrew's legs looked good.

As tense as Scott's day had been, he thought about Dr. D'Amato's. He could have canceled Andrew, but didn't. He had started early that morning, and now it was midnight. Dr. D'Amato's family would be asleep by the time he got home, and he had to start again early the next day. Scott asked Dr. D'Amato how he kept that pace.

"It's what I do," D'Amato said. That was his answer.

They decided to try removing the breathing tube again. This time, Scott remained in Andrew's room. He watched as they began to pull the tube free. Andrew gagged a little as it came out. There was a noise like air escaping from a half-knotted balloon. It was Andrew trying to breathe. Scott asked if he was all right.

His throat, they said, had tightened around the space where the tube had been, but air was getting through. To Scott it sounded unsustainable. He assumed they would reintubate him, but they didn't. They put on an oxygen mask and watched the monitors.

Rebecca came into the room. The sound alarmed her. It was like the breaths of someone about to give up. Then Andrew opened his eyes. He seemed to be trying to talk. Rebecca spoke to him.

"Andrew, what's the matter?"

The voice was so light and raspy you couldn't really hear it. You had to read lips.

"I don't want to be here," he mouthed.

Scott leaned near him. "Andrew. Dad's here. You're in the hospital. You've been very sick."

"I don't want to be here," he repeated.

Then he was out again. Rebecca certainly couldn't blame him for thinking that way.

His breathing did not improve. It went like that for hours. Each breath sounded as though it would be his last. Rebecca considered it inhumane to put Andrew through this. She kept asking if he should be reintubated. She found herself inhaling at the same time Andrew did, as if that would help him. Next to the bone scan, this was the worst day for her.

The doctors pointed out that he was holding his own. His oxygen was not dropping, and his sats were up. They checked his lungs by stethoscope, and picked up only minimal wheezing. That said the only problem was a constricted throat. Rebecca asked when this would end. All they could say was they would keep watching him.

Mike Day was there that night. He was alarmed by Andrew's gasping. He kept it together while there, but back home it got to him. It was the first time Mike had really fallen apart hard over this. He was relieved no one was around to see him.

Rebecca remained at Andrew's bedside, feeling he needed her there. She rubbed his stomach. It was a long night. It took three days before the gasping noise subsided.

Chapter 10

"We need to talk about what happened to you . . ."

D r. Pamela Feuer was the fourth intensivist. Her job, she concluded, would be to wake Andrew up. His kidneys were still shut down, his heart and lungs stressed, his wounds in need of daily debriding, but she thought Andrew needed to get moving, interact with his family. She had talked about it with Dr. Snelling, who agreed. This was the start of his fourth week. "Enough of this pall," Linda Snelling had said.

Dr. Snelling had found that patients with support got better more quickly. She'd heard the opposite often: "He just decided he was going to die." And did. The way Snelling figured it, if you can decide you're going to die, you can decide you're not going to. It was time to let this little boy see everyone pulling for him.

Slowly, Dr. Feuer began to dial down Andrew's sedation.

Andrew lifted his legs and brought them hard onto the bed. Both were in big, heavy casts. Rebecca found it startling. She wondered if he was in pain. He did it again. He tried to move his left arm, but it was secured by restraints to protect a main line. Rebecca asked a nurse if he was all right.

Yes. He was more physical than they'd expected, but this was the process.

. . .

Scott was nervous about Andrew waking up. It meant they would have to tell him. It would be another whole episode they were going to have to go through. He also worried about mental damage. At one point they had asked Dr. Morin about it, and she could not guarantee Andrew would be the same kid. Morin had not wanted to discourage Rebecca and Scott, but had said that yes, there were many small ways the brain could have been affected.

Andrew continued to lift and strike his legs against the mattress. Janice Costello, one of Rebecca's sisters, was visiting when he began doing this.

"Uh-oh," she said.

The parents were at the foot of his bed.

"Jan, what's the matter?"

"Look."

Rebecca came around. There was a widening pool of blood on the sheet beneath Andrew. The dialysis catheter that cycled blood back into his body had popped out of his right groin. It was a big tube held in with stitches, but his thrashing had dislodged it. Blood was pumping from the tube.

"Oh my God," said a nurse. She turned off the machine, but blood kept coming from his leg. She called for assistance. Several times she used the word *stat*. Dr. Feuer came in and put both hands atop the wound. She leaned over Andrew with straight elbows. It seemed she was using most of her body weight. Rebecca looked at the monitors. His heart rate was up and his pressure down. More people came into the room.

"I need platelets, stat," said Dr. Feuer.

Rebecca had not heard them order blood with such urgency since the first days. Within a minute they had started a drip. Rebecca stepped back from the bed, not wanting to get in everyone's hair. It couldn't be good, she thought, to bleed so much you need an emergency transfusion. Dr. Feuer kept the pressure on the leg. Rebecca could tell she was concerned. It took fifteen minutes for the vein to clot off. It took another hour to stabilize Andrew. It was ER stuff again, a bolus of this, a drip of that, careful adjustments while watching the monitor.

Man, Rebecca was thinking, *I thought this was over. I thought we were out of the woods.*

Dr. Feuer weighed whether to put the tube back in. It seemed necessary, since Andrew's kidneys were not functioning. A few days before, Dr. Snelling had attempted a trial, turning the machine off for several hours. It didn't work. On the other hand, because of its thickness, reinserting the tube would be a surgical procedure, complete with anesthesia. That would set Andrew back. He was breathing on his own, and sedating him more deeply could hamper that. It was a hard call.

Dr. Feuer met with Scott and Rebecca in the consultation room. Having just picked up service the day before from Dr. Snelling, this was Feuer's first real sit-down with the Batesons. She told them she wanted to leave the tube out for the time being. Her hope was that his kidneys might resume function on their own. There were risks of fluid and toxin buildup, but maybe Andrew's kidneys had gotten lazy. Why should they work, as long as something else was doing the job for them? This could jolt them back to life. Were the parents comfortable with that?

A week before, Rebecca had spoken to the kidney doctor. He was concerned that Andrew had yet to get any function back. Rebecca had asked what would happen if he didn't soon. Worst case, the doctor said, you're looking at a lifetime of dialysis; but they would cross that bridge when they had to. Rebecca told Dr. Feuer, "Yes, let's try it."

They watched his levels of BUN—blood urea nitrogen—and his creatinine. Those were the telltale signs of kidney function. The hope was that they would come down. After several hours, they had not. They continued testing through the night. Rebecca and Scott grew discouraged.

Late the next morning Dr. Feuer sat down with them. She had just gotten back the latest readings.

"Guess what?" she said. "His levels are lower. Can you believe it?"

They weren't a lot lower. Instead of being thirteen times the normal level, one number was twelve times. But at least it was the right direction. Later in the day, Andrew's kidneys stopped working again. His blood pressure went up, and they had to restart medication to control it. Dr. Feuer chose to hold course. Over the next days things gradually improved. No one knew if Andrew's kidneys would come all the way back, but he had turned a big corner.

Andrew grew more and more restless. He moved around, looked irritable, and grimaced. His eyes would flutter. From time to time he pulled an IV out. It wasn't anything to laugh about, but Rebecca told the nurses it was the kind of child Andrew was; he could be quite uncooperative.

The Batesons had gone outside the hospital entrance for air. A half dozen family members were with them. It was the evening of July 27, a Sunday. They had been in the hospital for twenty-three days. A friend who had been visiting upstairs came out.

"Andrew's awake," he said.

Everyone took the stairs, not wanting to wait for the elevator. Rebecca and Scott put on yellow precautions gowns without tying the backs and went in. Andrew's eyes were wide, like he had just had a weird dream. He did not seem drowsy. He had gone right from coma to awake.

"Hey, bud," Rebecca said. "How are you?"

She leaned down and pulled him to her. He squeezed back slightly with one arm, but was too weak to lift the other.

"Mom and Dad have been here the whole time," said Rebecca. "We haven't left you." Clearly, he was unaware of his legs. All Scott could think was, "Wow, Andrew's back." Word got around the unit. Nurses and residents came in. All the grown-ups wanted to say hello.

Andrew looked from face to face but was unable to talk. More people crowded around. It reminded Rebecca of that scene at the end of *The Wizard of Oz* when Dorothy wakes up.

The last thing Andrew had said before being put under was, "I'm thirsty." Now he formed those same words. Rebecca asked if he wanted a Popsicle. The nurses had some in a refrigerator for when kids were dehydrated; they said it would be okay. Rebecca touched it to his lips. To Scott, that was one good sight, Andrew licking that Popsicle. He couldn't swallow much, his throat being too tight.

Andrew grew tired and fell back asleep. He was in and out over the next day. He wasn't able to sit up or talk. He tried, but nothing came out. His vocal cords weren't there yet. There were dark circles beneath Andrew's eyes, and his skin had a gray cast. His face was disfigured by recovering purpura lesions. The doctors told the Batesons it would take time.

Someone told Andrew to stick out his tongue for the doctor. He did so, and when he got a reaction he kept doing it. Everyone got a kick out of that, but something bothered Rebecca. It was too exaggerated. When Andrew smiled, it was all teeth. That, too, troubled her. It wasn't quite right. At times he acted delirious. That added to Rebecca's concern. Was it the medication? Or some sort of brain damage? Scott picked up on it too. He thought of what Andrew's system had been through. If his legs were starved of oxygen, mightn't his brain have been?

Dr. Feuer tried to reassure the Batesons. When a child was on high doses of sedatives for a long time, it changed the chemicals of the brain. Kids had hallucinations and abnormal movements. They had odd emotional reactions. The parents asked if damage was possible.

Yes, but remotely.

The Batesons read Andrew's every gesture. This was the point of finding out where Andrew was.

One of the first words he used was "green." That was the kind of Popsicle he asked for. "Why green?" Rebecca asked. "Nobody wants green. Everybody wants cherry." Andrew wanted green. Visitors heard about this and the nurses' freezer was soon stuffed with boxes of green Popsicles.

Andrew was unconscious less often. He remained physically weak, his voice a rasp, but each day he became more appropriate in his responses. The doctors were confident it had not affected his brain.

Nurses told Scott and Rebecca it would be good to get Andrew's clock back in sync. After the visitors left they dimmed the lights. They used a small sponge to brush his teeth, just to get that ritual back in place. Such things gave them a feeling of life beginning again.

At bedtime Rebecca recited a familiar prayer to Andrew.

"Now I lay me down to sleep.

"I pray the Lord my soul to keep."

At that point, she gave it a new twist:

"Angels watch me through the night

"And wake me with the morning light."

She had learned it, of course, with a different ending: "If I die before I wake, I pray the Lord my soul to take." Rebecca didn't like that version. She had never liked it. She certainly wasn't going to say it that way now.

Andrew's legs remained in big casts, usually under the sheets. He never asked about them. He didn't look down, since he couldn't lift his head. He seemed to assume they were still there. Scott began to focus on telling Andrew. The idea was a huge mountain to him. Most of the PICU staff thought the same way; everyone was anxious about the approach of that moment.

The Batesons talked with different people about how to say it. No one was able to lay out exact words for them; there was no instruction book. "You'll find a way," friends told them. "You're good parents. It'll come to you." The psychiatrists and social workers offered to help, even to be there, but in the end Scott and Rebecca knew it was on them.

Rebecca sat with Cindy Day in the family room. She was low. "How is he going to look at us that we allowed this to happen to him?"

Cindy didn't want to give false assurances. It touched on her own fears as a mother. Your children expected you to protect them. She wasn't sure what to say.

There was a big coffee table in the corner of the room. Rebecca thought how much she wanted to crawl under it. She didn't want anyone to find her until it was over. That was how the whole thing left her feeling: as if she wanted to disappear into a crevice.

Scott knew they had to tell Andrew soon; it would be wrong for Andrew to figure it out by himself. On the other hand, he feared this would change Andrew. You didn't go through something like that and stay the same kid. Scott kept having memories of Andrew coming down the sidewalk on Rollerblades with his sister and friends. The memories were always of a sunny spring-summer day. He could visualize it in detail.

Rebecca had similar pictures in her head: what a wild skier Andrew had been. His first time on a slope he got off the chairlift, gave a little war whoop, and off he went. He was five years old. Rebecca called for him to slow down, but he kept going. He loved that feeling of speed. He got mad whenever she or Scott stopped him.

Late evening Scott and Rebecca walked into Andrew's room. Their daughter, Erin, went in too. They shut the door. It was just the four of them. The nurses could tell this was the moment. Andrew had already asked about the casts, so it was time. It was July 31, a

Thursday, four days after he had woken up. Lynn Cavaliero watched with Suzanne Kiniry. "How do people get through this?" Suzanne said to Lynn. "How do they do this?" Lynn had no answer.

Andrew was watching television. He was too weak to sit up, but seemed cheerful. "Honey," Rebecca said, "we really need to talk about what happened to you." The parents were on either side of the bed.

"You remember that you were very, very sick," Rebecca said, "but you're getting better." She tried not to sound depressed. If Mom acted like it was all right, maybe Andrew would take that in.

"Well, you were very sick, honey—your whole body was very sick. You're getting better but your legs didn't get better, so the doctors had to take them off. If they didn't, hon, you wouldn't have gotten better. But we're going to get you new legs."

Andrew started to cry. There was no "Let me see." Or "What do you mean they're not there?" That told her he had suspected something; it had sunk in that quickly. Andrew asked why they did it. He was crying hard now.

"They had to take your old legs because they were very sick," Rebecca said.

Scott paced. "I knew we shouldn't have done this now," he said.

Rebecca told him there was no good time.

Scott kept pacing. It was almost too much for him. Erin began to cry. It occurred to Rebecca it was the first time she had done so since Andrew fell ill.

Rebecca kept assuring Andrew that they would get new legs.

"I want my old legs back, Mommy." He was crying and crying.

"You can't, hon," Rebecca said. "They won't work anymore."

One reason she held her answers short was to keep from sobbing herself. There was a big lump in her throat. Rebecca believed it had taken all of the last five weeks to build herself up for this moment.

After a while Andrew asked a different kind of question.

Would he ever be able to walk again?

"Oh yeah," Rebecca said. "I've heard stories of kids who've done all kinds of things."

"Will I be able to run?"

"It's going to take some work, but I don't see why you can't be like those other kids."

He asked how he would ride his Harley bike.

"We'll figure out a way," Rebecca said. Six-year-olds, she knew, believed everything their parents said, so she didn't want to over-promise. That could lose his trust down the road.

Then he returned to wanting his own legs back. He asked where they were.

Rebecca said she didn't know.

Most of the time, he cried. It went on like that for hours.

Around midnight, it got quiet. The television was tuned to Nick-elodeon. *I Love Lucy* was playing. For a few minutes Andrew watched it. It struck Scott that this was the first time just the four of them had been alone together. There was something comforting about that. Andrew asked if he would be able to go back to his school.

Yes, of course, hon.

By 1 A.M. or so, he was mostly gazing at the television.

Scott couldn't tell whether Andrew had calmed down or had drawn into himself.

"But how will I be able to ride my bike?"

"We'll work on that, honey."

Rebecca felt a small bit of relief. Telling Andrew had been such a looming cloud. She had thought he would be angry with them for letting the doctors do this. She would have had no answer if he had accused her of that. It never came up, though. She also had expected him to withdraw into silence. Maybe, she thought, all those questions were good. At least he was facing it enough to try figuring it out.

Around 4 A.M., Andrew fell asleep. Erin did too. She dozed on the lower half of Andrew's bed. Scott and Rebecca settled into the two vinyl chairs, neither of which was comfortable, but they did the job. The previous hour or so, Andrew had stopped crying. He was even playing with his sister, some game involving Beanie Babies. There were tons of them in the room. The whole ledge behind the bed was full of stuffed animals.

Scott remained tense. He assumed that Andrew would be despondent when he awoke, and get worse each day. It was such an impossible weight on a little guy. He was not yet seven. Scott considered it the start of a long, bad road. The thought of it was a hurt deep in his chest.

Andrew woke up. Scott asked if he wanted to watch television.

"Yeah." He seemed interested. It was just after dawn.

How about this station, Andrew?

Yeah, fine. He was going along normally, like nothing had happened. It continued like that all morning. Rebecca wondered if there was some odd dynamic going on. Maybe Andrew had repressed it, like people do after a trauma. Maybe he thought it had been a dream or something.

A nurse and technician came into the room.

"Do they know about my legs, Mommy?" said Andrew.

"Yeah, honey, they do."

"Okay, Mommy."

Scott was surprised. Andrew seemed so relaxed it made you feel better. It was just one morning, though.

Midday, Andrew brought it up again. He asked why they had to take his legs off. Rebecca told him how he wouldn't have gotten better if the doctors didn't.

"Oh."

That was all he said.

The day's visitors began to show up. As each left, another arrived. Most brought gifts. Scott and Rebecca opened them, since Andrew could not use his hands. All along, the staff continued their work. There was also the TV. Andrew got to have a Popsicle whenever he wanted. He was one busy kid. Scott felt that helped.

That night Erin and Andrew lay side by side, watching television. To Scott, Andrew seemed to be having an okay time, just hanging out. Scott liked these moments without visitors. It had been a long time since they were just a family. If they could catch an hour when the nurses wouldn't have to do something, that was the best; no one but them in the room. Even if they were zoned out on TV, no one talking, that was fine. It felt good for it to be only the four of them. Still, every time Scott glanced at Andrew he couldn't get his mind off what was happening.

Erin now came to the hospital regularly. She and Andrew would lie on the bed, watching TV together. Scott considered it a highlight of Andrew's day. You could see that brother-sister closeness. The old Andrew came out more when Erin was there. Once she brought a jar of hermit crabs from the beach, complete with rocks and seaweed. The two set up the throw-up basin as a temporary hermit crab zoo.

Scott looked out the window. It was cloudy and windy outdoors. It began to rain. It was late afternoon, and dark. The door was closed and Andrew was sleeping. There were no nurses or technicians in the room. Everything felt serene. It was like one of those rainy days where you don't want to get out of bed and don't have to.

They had a portable cassette player in the room. They had put in *Evening Passages* by Ed Van Fleet. It was soothing music. The cuts included "Twilight Path" and "Baby's Lullaby." Someone knocked lightly on the door. "May I come in?" It was one of the religious clergy at the hospital, a nun named Sister Perpetua. She would visit from time to time. She said, "I can feel the peace in here."

Scott didn't try to fool himself into thinking everything was fine, but it was okay for this moment. He reached over to rub Andrew's chest and stomach. He sat there and listened to the rain.

"Daddy," Andrew said. "Could you get the statue behind me?" He was talking about the plaster figure of Jesus they had brought to the hospital from their home. Scott carried it to the bed. Andrew touched its face. He said something about it looking alive. Then he said, "You can put it back."

Later Rebecca said to Scott, "How did he know that was even back there?" It was out of Andrew's view, and he could not turn around. There were no mirrors to reflect it, and no one had mentioned it. Scott considered the moment a sign. So did Father Ken, even though he wasn't a statue guy himself. How else could you explain Andrew being aware of it?

Rebecca had never known Andrew to be conscious of such things. In the past the only comment he had made on religion was that he didn't want to go to church. He was always a handful during Mass, paid no attention, "had" to go to the bathroom two or three times. When he was little he would toss his pacifier three pews forward so he could crawl after it. Rebecca once caught him dropping action figures into open handbags on the pew in front of them.

She and Andrew spent most of the time in the "crying room," a glassed-in space in the back of St. Pius. There were usually three or four kids in there, running around with their Cheerios and bottles as if at play group. The Mass was piped in, but there was usually so much noise you couldn't make it out. Erin left the crying room at age two and a half. Andrew remained there well into his fourth year, making him one of the elder residents. Rebecca watched other families come and go. Sometimes she tried venturing out, but it seldom worked. Andrew was incapable of whispering. Once Scott carried him forward for communion. When Scott took just the bread, no wine, Andrew loudly asked, "What about a drink, Dad?" Back to the crying room.

But now Andrew wanted to see a religious statue. Another time he told Father Ken his hands and legs had been hurt like Jesus. Rebecca found it surprising that he was aware of such things, even a bit weird. It made her wonder whether he had been to a different place. It was compelling in a way, but also gave her the creeps.

Rebecca had been unable to hold Andrew for a month. Finally, they were going to let her. It was a slow process. They had to make sure all the IVs stayed attached. Carefully, two nurses and Scott lifted him from the hospital bed. Rebecca sat with pillows on either side of her to help cushion him.

It had been a week since the operation. Andrew's legs were still in casts. Rebecca did not think about that at the moment. Her focus was on having her son in her arms. The separation had at times left her feeling less than a mother. They placed Andrew in her lap.

He was more fragile than she expected. His head flopped like that of a newborn. She was afraid he might bend the wrong way, or that she would squeeze him too tight. He had burns everywhere. Rebecca sat rigidly, worried about dislodging the tubes. It was not the comforting moment she had anticipated. After a few minutes she told the nurses it wasn't working. Carefully they transferred him back to the bed.

Dr. Ginger Manzo, from psychiatry, stopped by the room. A few of Andrew's friends were visiting. They were telling a story where each person added onto it. When it was Andrew's turn he couldn't come up with anything and began to cry. He seemed frustrated at not being able to focus.

Dr. Kleinman came back on duty. The Batesons had been there long enough to go through the full cycle of intensivists. Kleinman told them, "Wouldn't it be neat if we can get him moved up to the fifth floor?" The fifth was a normal floor, a big step up for pediatric ICU patients.

Kleinman's first exam found Andrew more emaciated than she'd expected. He needed everything done for him. His hands were limited, and it was unclear how much use he would regain there. Dr. Kleinman also found him depressed. He seemed all right with his parents, but he didn't want to interact with others. To Kleinman he was a sad, withdrawn child. She wasn't sure the parents saw that side of him. She chose not to tell the Batesons how different Andrew appeared to the staff.

As the days progressed, she was able to remove some of his lines. On August 6, the day before Dr. Kleinman's week ended, she sat down with the Batesons in the consultation room.

"You know what, guys," she said. "I think we're going to move Andrew." They would do it the next day. She had already put in the paperwork. Kleinman did not say it out loud, but part of her hope was to give his mood a helpful push.

Nurses from the fifth floor came down with an extra gurney for the family's personal things. "Just load it up," they told Scott and Rebecca. The Batesons began to do so. They piled on posters, cards, stuffed animals, and little plaques. *You don't realize*, Rebecca thought, *just how much stuff you collect in a few short weeks.*

It was a good feeling, leaving, but Scott found it a little sad. This was the staff who had pulled Andrew through. They all came to see him off. It was a real farewell thing. Everyone said they would miss him. Once upstairs, Scott sized up the new room. He looked out the window. It wasn't comfortable yet. Pretty odd, he thought, that the intensive care unit, the saddest place in the hospital, had come to feel like home.

Dr. Kleinman watched as they wheeled Andrew toward the elevators. What came next, she suspected, was going to be tougher than the Batesons realized. Rehabilitation was a lot to ask of such a sick little guy. His spirit seemed dulled. It worried her. There was just no energy there.

As they told him good-bye, Suzanne Kiniry and Lynn Cavaliero were unsure about Andrew too. Suzanne thought he had slipped into a depression. Lynn guessed that he was angry. He wouldn't make eye contact with anyone but his parents. When he did speak to the staff, it was seldom more than a word or two. Suzanne had tried to draw him out, but he just stared at the corner of his room. She didn't blame him. Maybe it was the one thing he could control.

Chapter 11

"I'll be able to do stuff like Erin?"

Casey Little and Lori LaFrance had worked with plenty of trauma kids—head injuries, cancer, burns—but never a patient without legs, and this frail. Those in Hasbro's rehabilitation department could remember few children with such a severity of need.

Now that Andrew Bateson had been moved to the fifth floor, the rehab therapists were the most frequent staffers in his room. You could often hear them coming; they wore nylon jogging suits, which made a swishing sound as they walked. The suits were for floor work, and also for times when children might get sick on them. They all had stories of cooing at babies who would suddenly respond that way.

Scott looked out the window of Andrew's new room. *Wow,* he thought, *we're a long way up.* The view was different from the second floor. Things also felt more relaxed on the fifth. During much of the day Andrew watched videos or whatever was on TV. That gave Scott time to think about things. He doubted life would ever be normal again. He wasn't sure how it could be.

Casey and Lori asked the docs to let them try placing Andrew in a wheelchair. Children, they knew, could lose 20 percent of their strength each week they remained bedridden. The longer Andrew lay there, the more debilitated he became. The two positioned a reclining wheelchair next to him. This would be a big test. Lori lifted Andrew's bottom half, Casey his top. They had to be careful of all the skin-compromised areas. They lowered him into the seat.

"Look at you, Andrew," Lori said. "You look great." Andrew was sitting on his own. To Scott that was one nice sight. Then Andrew complained of back pain and slouched like a rag doll. He couldn't support himself. It blew Scott's mind how weak Andrew was. It took them a week to get Andrew up to a forty-five-degree recline. Even then, he would slouch. Scott wondered if his son would ever regain his normal strength.

Several times a day the therapists came to the room to range Andrew's limbs. He could not lift them himself. To Rebecca, it looked as though Casey and Lori were moving the arms of a child who was asleep. She couldn't see how that would count for exercise, but she supposed they had to start somewhere.

Scott and Rebecca stood in the hallway with Dr. D'Amato. He had just finished examining Andrew. The parents were somewhat upbeat, with their son awake and out of bed. D'Amato talked about Andrew's legs, then changed the subject. He hated to bring more bad news, but he was worried about Andrew's hands. They had curled into rigid claws. Because of the bandages it hadn't been that obvious to Scott, but yes, Andrew's hands had locked in a way that reminded him of children with cerebral palsy. Dr. D'Amato said it was a condition called Volkmann's contracture.

What caused it?

When the meningococcemia cut off oxygen, he explained, it killed nerves and tendons. The month-long coma, by immobilizing his hands, made the damage worse. D'Amato thought Andrew would have permanent deficits. Other doctors had warned of this, but D'Amato's prognosis was more worrisome. He was an orthopedic surgeon. He knew bones and muscles.

Mightn't Andrew's fingers just be frozen from inactivity? A temporary thing?

Years before, said D'Amato, he had done work in countries where there had been earthquakes. He had treated children trapped under rubble. Once nerves and tendons scarred up and then atrophied, the result was often permanent. D'Amato had asked the therapists to be aggressive, but he did not want Scott and Rebecca to hope for too much. Scott's first thought was *Here we go again.*

Scott watched closely as Casey Little unbandaged Andrew's hands. One by one, she took a curled finger and bent back the tip a fraction. Then she went to the next. Casey got almost no movement out of them. The process demanded a lot of patience.

Scott and Rebecca asked what the two therapists thought would happen in time. Andrew would at least be able to feed himself, wouldn't he?

"We'll work our best to get there," Lori said. She had learned you didn't speculate.

Scott asked if he could try. Carefully, with Casey's guidance, he took the last section of Andrew's index finger. It felt like rigor mortis had set in; at least he assumed that would be the feel of a hand in that condition. The other fingers felt the same. When the session was done, there had been no progress.

Would this be all right to do on his own?

Yes, Casey said, but carefully. Bend his fingers too far, and it would damage tendons. That would make the condition worse.

That afternoon Scott worked each finger. It did not go well. Both hands were like wooden claws. And Andrew complained throughout.

Rebecca was next to them. "Don't stretch them too far back," she said.

After a few minutes Scott said, "Look, this one does move a little."

"Be careful, Scott."

...

He continued the exercises three times a day, a half hour per session. Sometimes he did it at 1 or 2 A.M. It was not a big sacrifice, as Scott wasn't sleeping anyway. Both hands had extensive skin lesions. The end of Andrew's index finger was almost black. At one point, during regular therapy, the top half inch of it came off. The fingertip, including much of the nail area, just fell away. That was the kind of damage Andrew had.

After three or four days, Andrew's fingers still could barely be moved. It demoralized Scott. He suspected the doctors were right; perhaps the hands wouldn't come back. Then Scott caught himself. It didn't help to think like that. The least he could do was stay at it for Andrew. Besides, the exercises helped Scott's head. It was the first time he was able to actually do something. The thing that got him down was just watching. That felt helpless to him.

Rebecca had a lot of respect for the way Scott hung in there on Andrew's hands. She wasn't sure she could have done it, but Scott didn't flag. It was like a mission to him. As husband and wife, though, they still had their issues; the connection just wasn't there.

Some family members invited Dr. Monica Kleinmen to a fundraiser for the Batesons at St. Pius. On the way there, Kleinman pictured fifty people in a church hall. There were 400.

Rebecca gave an update on Andrew's condition. Then she said she wanted to make a special mention. It's not often, Rebecca said, that you get to publicly thank the person who saved your child's life. She asked Dr. Kleinman to stand. The crowd got to its feet and gave her a loud ovation. It took Kleinman by surprise, as she really didn't know any of these people. The applause went on so long she began to feel awkward.

Afterward, person after person came up to her. The night turned into a whole string of thank-yous. It was an emotional moment for Dr. Kleinman, who had never experienced such a display of gratitude. Doctors, she thought, seldom get to see so directly the impact of their work.

· · ·

The fund-raiser ended after midnight. As Scott and Rebecca were preparing to leave, the hospital called. Scott took it. It was a nurse.

"It's not an emergency call," she said off the top, "but I don't want you to be walking in tonight and saying, 'Oh God, what happened?'"

What did happen?

Somehow, Andrew's main line came out of his neck. He was fine now, but there was a lot of blood.

Scott's brother Jimmy and his wife, Lori, had been watching Andrew.

"Uncle Jimmy did it," said Andrew when his parents returned.

Jimmy looked at Scott, as if to say *It wasn't like that.*

Andrew had an impish look.

"What do you mean, buddy?" asked Scott.

"Uncle Jimmy. He was moving me and it fell out."

Sometimes Andrew slid down from his pillow, and it was routine for an adult to slide him back up. Jimmy nodded. Yes, he had been doing that, and maybe play-wrestling with Andrew a bit, but—

"Uncle Jimmy did it," Andrew said again. He was giving his uncle up. It was that lighter side of Andrew. He liked to fool with people.

Jimmy had always gotten a kick out of Andrew. He wasn't a shy kid, that was for sure. Once Andrew asked Jimmy why he smoked. Everything with Andrew was "why."

"I don't know," said Uncle Jimmy. "Just a bad habit."

Andrew said that seemed stupid, didn't it?

There was nothing Jimmy could say to defend himself. It was funny to get scolded by so young a child. But that was Andrew. Whatever was on his mind, you were going to hear it.

Scott hoped it was the beginning of Andrew getting playful again. Most of the time he seemed pretty low.

· · ·

There was only one chair in Andrew's fifth-floor hospital room. Sometimes, when it was taken, Rebecca would sit in the wheelchair. One night she fell asleep in it, leaning over with her head against the mattress. At 2 A.M., she was roused by Andrew yelling. A nurse had come in to start a procedure on him, one Rebecca thought could have waited. She got angry, asking why the nurse would just start in without telling the parents.

"Oh, well, I'm very sorry," she said.

"You tell me what you're going to do to him," said Rebecca. "We've been aware of what's been going on." From now on, she said, things needed to be discussed with them in advance.

"Oh. I'm very sorry."

Later, Rebecca realized it was unfair to have attacked the nurse that way. Things were getting to her. The fifth floor was an adjustment.

A nurse announced that visiting hours were over. It was 8 P.M., time to say good-bye.

"Mommy," Erin whispered, "I don't want to." Could she please stay, like in the PICU room?

There were different rules on the fifth floor. Young siblings weren't allowed to sleep in the room.

Okay, Rebecca told Erin. But if she got caught they would have to take her to a neighbor's. At first Rebecca thought of hiding Erin in the shower, then chose to cover her with a blanket in the corner chair. Every time the door opened Rebecca sat up to block the nurse's view. That was how they got through the night.

Early the next morning a nurse came in and saw Erin asleep in the corner.

"Oh," said Rebecca. "She just got here."

A few days later, they tried it again. At 2 A.M., a nurse woke up Scott.

"You know, your daughter's not supposed to be here. I'm going to have to let the charge nurse know."

Scott didn't get too riled up about it. He was tired. He knew they had broken the rules. They would face whatever they had to face. As it turned out, no one came back that night to read them the riot act.

The next day Rebecca approached the charge nurse herself. "We've been here for almost six weeks," she said. "I have to think of my other child."

"You have to understand," said the nurse. "Some of the parents would use this as free baby-sitting. They'd be dropping kids here and taking off."

"You know we're not that kind of family."

The nurse was sorry. She couldn't make exceptions. If others found out, it could cause a problem.

Lynn Cavaliero got a call from the fifth floor. She was told she had to do something about Scott and Rebecca. They kept sneaking Erin in to spend the night. Although stationed in the PICU, where she had grown close with the Batesons, Lynn was on rotation covering the building as manager, so a problem like this was on her.

Lynn was tempted to explain how PICU nurses winked at the sleepover rule, but knew that wouldn't matter. The fifth floor was different. She went up to talk to Scott and Rebecca.

"This is hard for me to have this discussion," she said, "but there've been complaints."

"We're all just trying to be together," said Scott.

Lynn felt like a heel. She had been through so much with this family.

"Fine," she said. "Could we all just go on record that we talked?"

While he was in a coma, Andrew's stomach wasn't able to process even liquids, so he was fed protein by IV. After he awoke, they switched to a nasogastric feeding tube.

But they were even having problems with that. Usually he gave the supplement right back to them. They tried everything: warming it, feeding it slowly. Occasionally he kept it down, and everyone said they had solved it, but the next time it would come back up. The doctors said Andrew's digestive tract had been shut down so long it wasn't able to take anything. It was also irritated from medications. Rebecca suspected that his stomach was where he put a lot of his stress.

A few times they removed his NG tube and tried to feed him by mouth. He managed one or two bites, and that was it. He didn't want any more. He said he felt sick. His face was drawn, with dark circles under his eyes. Andrew remained at thirty-nine pounds, never gaining an ounce more. They called it "failure to thrive." Rebecca began to fear that Andrew would have to go on a G tube, surgically implanted in his stomach to bypass the esophagus. The doctors said it could come to that.

Some wondered if Andrew might have a blockage. Rebecca became convinced of it. They took him for an endoscopy. She hoped that was what they would find. At least it would give them something to fix. But there was just irritation. It was a disappointment.

The hospital had little red wagons with attached IV poles. Scott and Rebecca used one to take Andrew on a walk. They lined it with blankets and took him to the garden. It was his first time outside. Andrew quickly grew tired, and said he wanted to go back to bed.

They began to take regular walks. Scott and Rebecca liked to park him near the lobby windows so he could look out. Robin Vargas, their social worker, ran into them there. Andrew looked sad to her.

"How you doing, buddy?" she asked, trying to sound as upbeat as she could. He didn't want to talk.

"We're not too happy today," Rebecca explained.

Robin believed you needed to treat kids with the same respect as adults, so she walked on, giving him his space.

Occasionally, the Child Life Department put on outdoor barbecues for the kids. The Batesons wheeled Andrew down to one. Robin Vargas approached him. She asked how things were going.

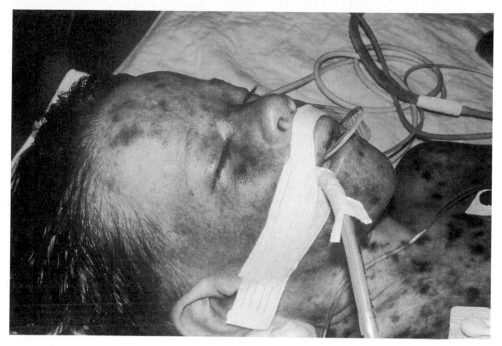

Within hours of reaching the hospital, Andrew Bateson was in a coma and on a ventilator, a victim of bacterial meningitis, one of the quickest-spreading infections known to medicine. Doctors gave him little chance for survival. (Providence Journal)

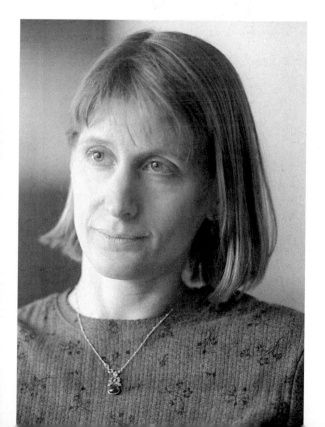

A surge in local cases of bacterial meningitis the previous year had left Dr. Monica Kleinman an expert on this otherwise rare disease. Andrew became her patient. (Providence Journal)

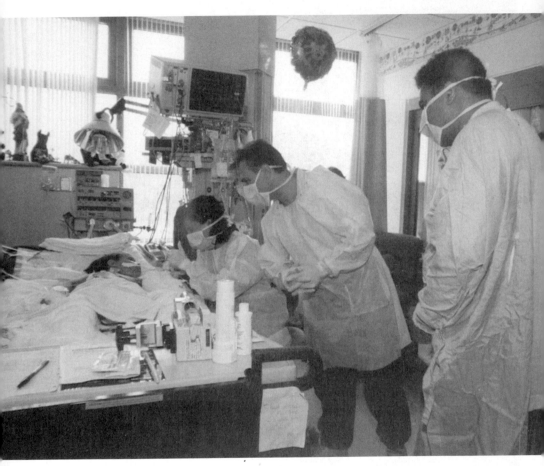

Rebecca and Scott Bateson spent almost every hour in full-precaution gowns at Andrew's bedside during his sixty-seven days in the hospital. On one of those days, Muhammed Ali came for a visit. (Family Photo)

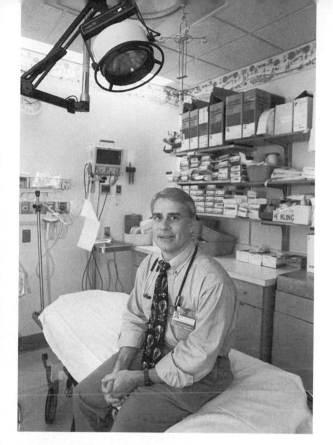

Jim Linakis was the attending physician at Hasbro Children's emergency department when Andrew arrived. Within seconds, Linakis knew he was looking at one of the most aggressive cases of bacterial meningitis he had ever seen. (Providence Journal)

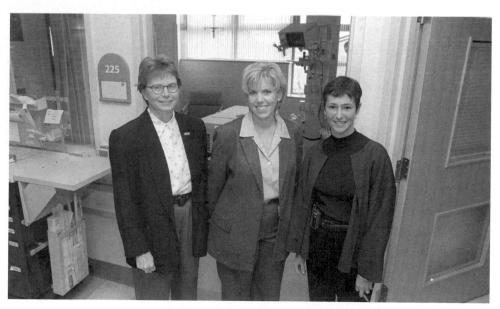

The four attending physicians at Pediatric Intensive Care did week-long rotations on the unit taking care of Andrew. Dr Kleinman's three colleagues were, from left, Dr. Linda Snelling, Dr. Pam Feuer, and Dr. Mindy Morin. (Providence Journal)

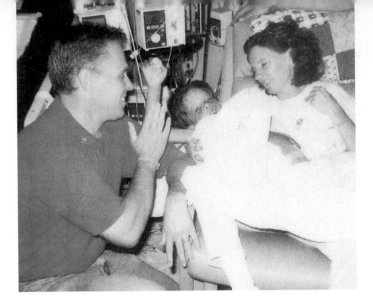

A month after entering the hospital, Rebecca was able to hold her son Andrew for the first time, as Scott knelt at their side. (Family Photo)

The bacterial meningitis left Andrew's body covered with the equivalent of third-degree burns. To prevent infection, Lori LaFrance and her colleagues had to spend long hours with Andrew in a whirlpool bath, scrubbing off the dead skin. (Providence Journal)

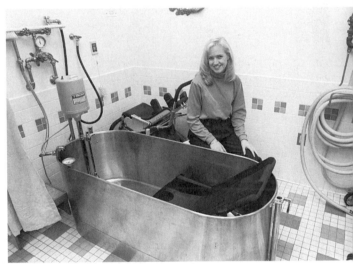

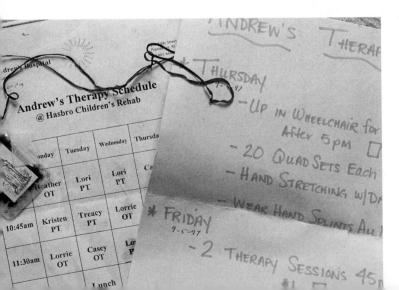

His parents placed cloth scapulars, including this one, below Andrew's knees before surgery, hoping for a miracle. (Providence Journal)

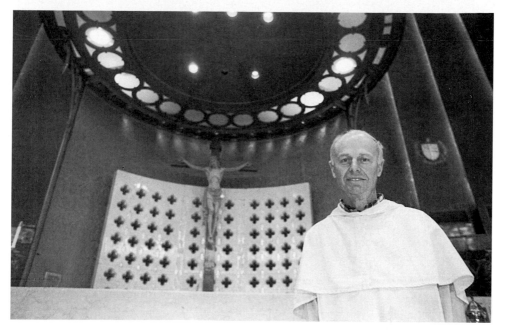

Father Ken Letoile, shown hear at St. Pius, where he served as pastor, said that in Andrew's hospital room he felt the presence of Jesus in a way that remains a singular experience in his priesthood. (Providence Journal)

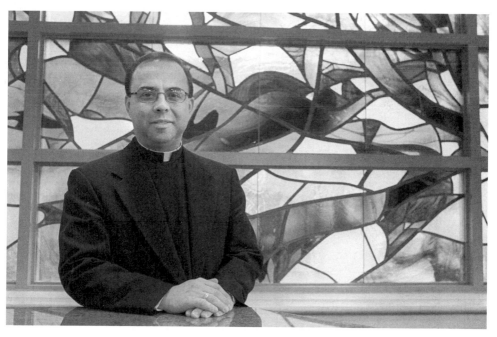

Father Joe Escobar, who sometimes ribbed other priests for being too "spiritual," was nevertheless convinced prayer made a tangible difference in Andrew's medical outcome. (Providence Journal)

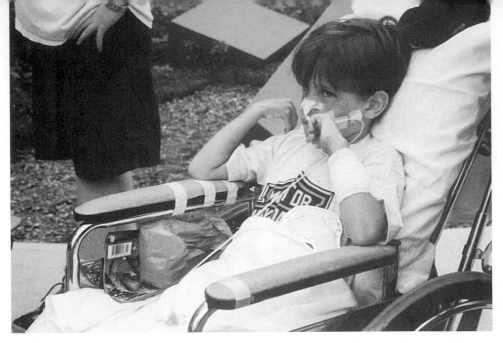

Andrew's doctors and therapists felt he was sinking into depression as he realized the toll of the illness. (Family Photo)

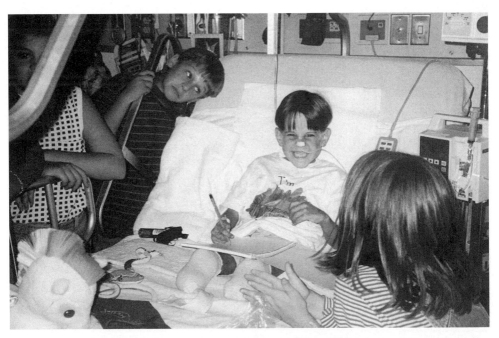

His parents were at first worried Andrew's friends would be afraid of approaching a boy who had just lost two legs. But children proved more comfortable in the hospital room than some adults, and Andrew was buoyed by their visits. (Providence Journal)

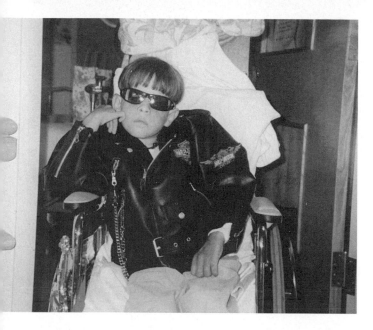

The Batesons' neighbor Joseph Mullen, a house painter who watches every cent, didn't think twice about spending $159 for a leather Harley jacket for Andrew. His caregivers felt Andrew's alter-ego personality—with jacket and shades—was a good coping mechanism for him.
(Providence Journal)

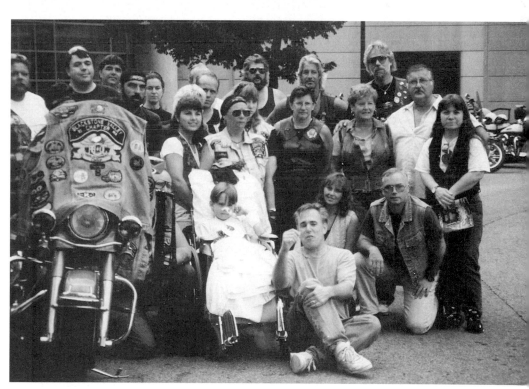

After word got out that a little boy in the hospital had a thing about motorcycles, a group of Harley bikers roared up and made Andrew an official member of their organization.
(Family Photo)

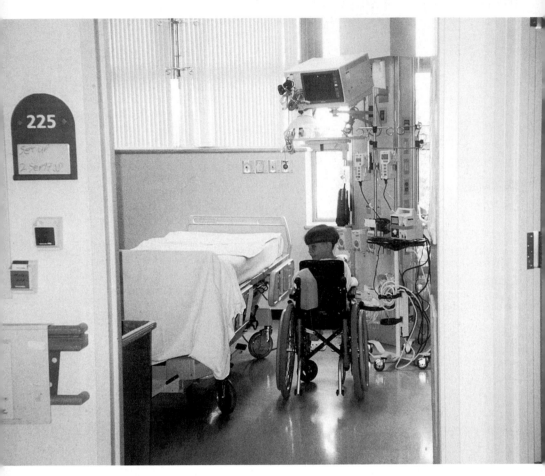

The Batesons were at last told they could take Andrew home, two months after he was hospitalized. On the way out, he stopped by the Pediatric Intensive Care unit to say goodbye to the room where his life had been saved. (Family Photo)

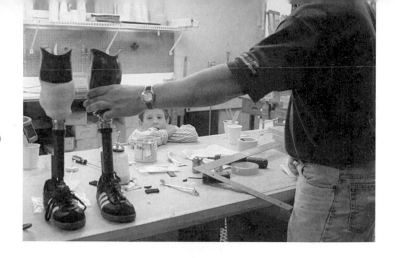

Andrew watches a prosthetic technician at Next Step put the finishing touches on his latest set of "fake legs." (Providence Journal)

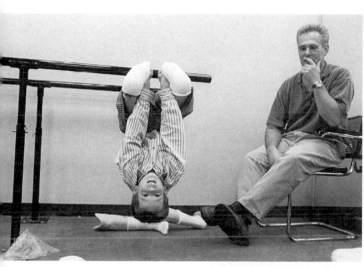

Scott Bateson looks on as his son clowns around while awaiting his new legs. Scott would often observe that Andrew seldom stopped moving. (Providence Journal)

Andrew tests out his new legs. The legs would soon be back in the shop for repairs after getting banged up from skating, biking, and running. "Boy," one of the prosthetic technicians said, "he really uses these." (Providence Journal)

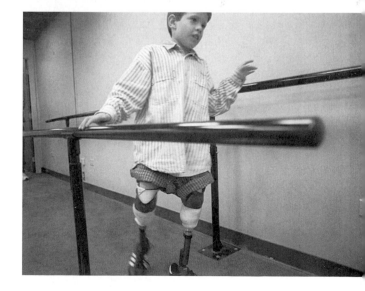

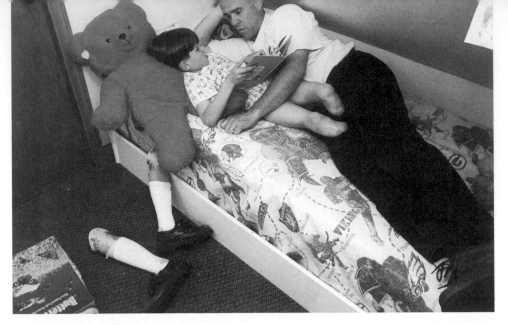

Andrew and his dad, back home at last. (Providence Journal)

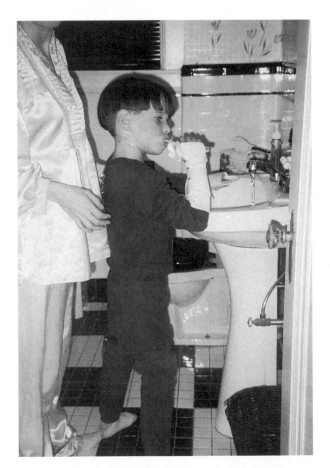

The disease had starved Andrew's hands of oxygen, leaving them badly damaged. Doctors doubted he would have full use of them again. He had to wear special splints at night to slowly stretch out his fingers. (Family Photo)

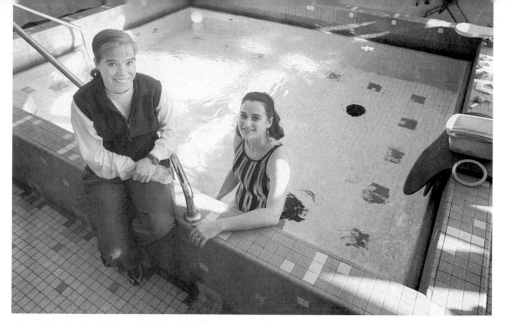

Casey Little and Kristen Montgomery were on the team that spent months teaching Andrew to walk and use his hands again. They often did exercises in the rehab pool at Hasbro Hospital. (Providence Journal)

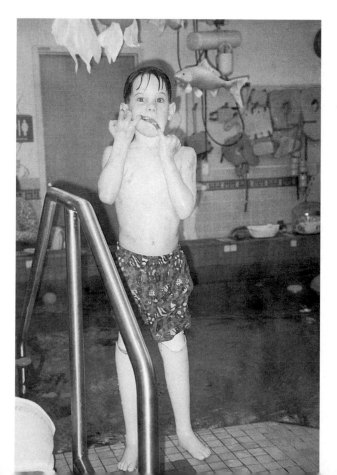

The rehab therapists found Andrew one of the most resistant patients they had ever worked with, and also one of the most impish. (Family Photo)

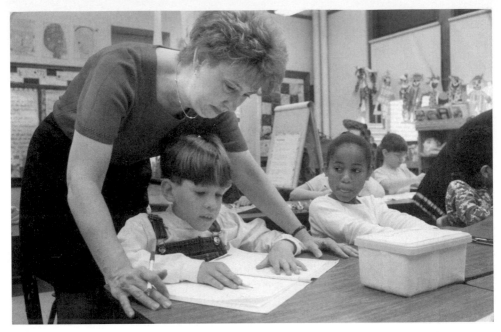

Meg Ford, Andrew's second-grade teacher, had lost her husband, Wayne, after a sixteen-year fight with cancer. Mrs. Ford felt that Andrew, like Wayne, was able to embrace life fully by focusing on what he had, rather than what he'd lost. (Providence Journal)

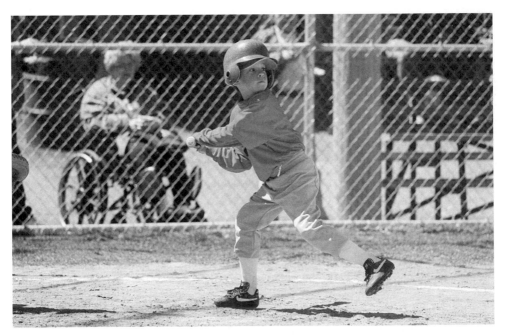

Andrew's parents worried Little League would prove too strenuous for a child without legs. It was the opposite: Andrew actually chose to move on to other sports because baseball had too much waiting time between plays. (Providence Journal)

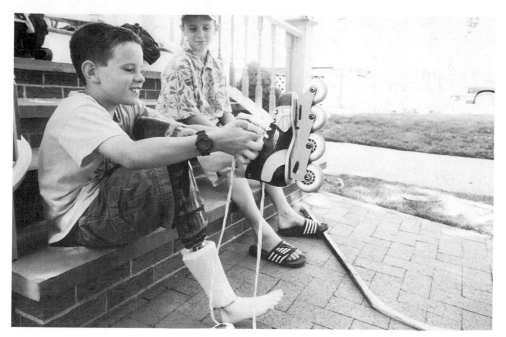

Rebecca discouraged Andrew from trying to Rollerblade again. She felt it would be too diffi-cult for a bilateral amputee. Andrew did not listen to her. (Family Photo)

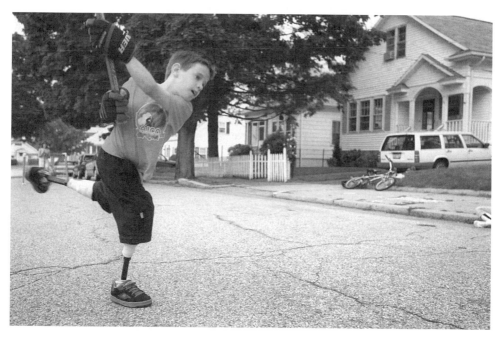

Andrew used the street in front of his white, tree-shaded home for biking, skating, or just practicing his slapshot. The white picket fence behind him is the one he held on to hour after hour while teaching himself to Rollerblade. (Providence Journal)

For much of his first season, no one in Andrew's ice hockey league knew he was skating on prosthetic legs. When Andrew's coach was eventually told, he said to Scott, "That kid has more guts than anyone I've ever seen on the ice."
(Providence Journal)

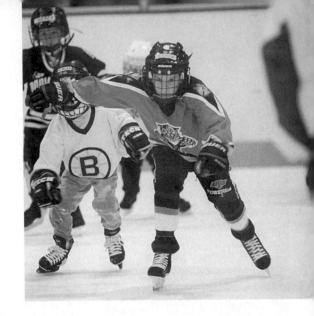

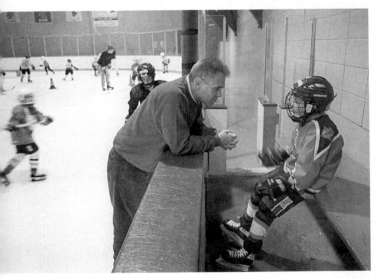

Andrew was frustrated on the ice when, after frequent falls, he couldn't stand back up without his dad's help. Eventually, Scott decided to pretend he didn't see, forcing Andrew to learn to get up on his own.
(Providence Journal)

Ice hockey quickly became Andrew's favorite sport.
(Providence Journal)

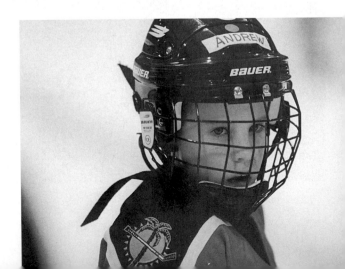

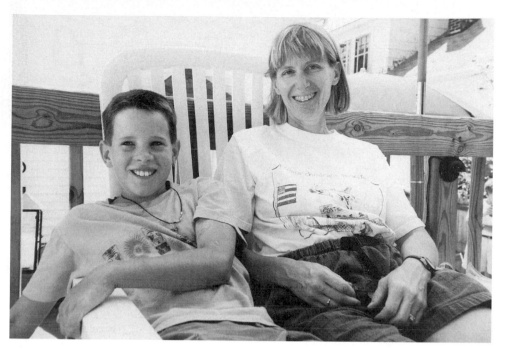

Dr. Monica Kleinman came to visit her patient after he was fully active again. She took a photograph of Andrew on Rollerblades and later displayed it in her new office at Boston Children's to remind herself why she does what she does. (Family Photo)

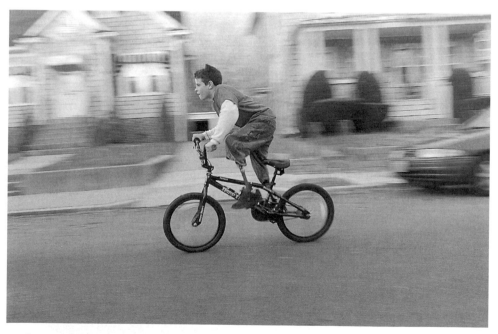

Andrew on his way to trying to "catch air" off a curb. (Family Photo)

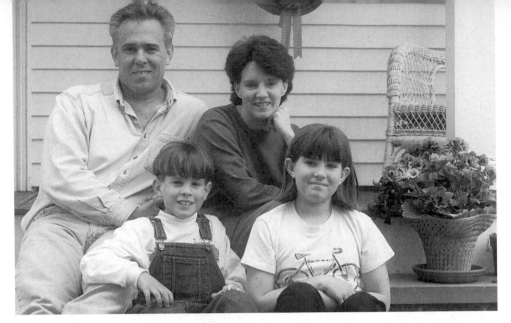

Scott and Rebecca Bateson and their children, Andrew and Erin, in the summer of 1999, two years after Andrew almost died from bacterial meningitis. (Family Photo)

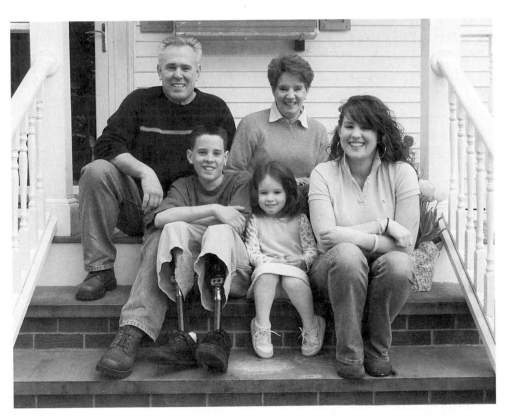

The Bateson family in 2005, along with their new addition, Abigail Faith. (Family Photo)

Andrew shrugged. He looked really down. He wanted to go back inside. He was still at that depressed place.

On August 14, the doctors took Andrew's leg casts off. His parents used a sheet to block his view. He said he wasn't ready to look at his legs. Frankly, Scott and Rebecca weren't either. Most of the time his pajamas covered them.

The therapists wanted to start desensitizing the skin there so they could try prosthetics. Andrew wouldn't cooperate. He couldn't handle anything touching his legs, not even a washcloth. He was very dramatic about it. Sometimes he yelled. They told him they had to do this if he was to get new legs. Andrew said he didn't want new legs, he just wanted to go home.

Casey and Lori brought up a box of small plastic dinosaurs. They asked Andrew to pick them up one at a time and put them in a second box. The idea was to get him using his hands again. It didn't go well. The plastic dinosaurs slipped out as he tried to lift them. It made Scott think of that arcade game where children lower a flimsy metal claw over a pile of toys and never get anything.

The therapists brought a bucket of dried rice. They told Andrew there were dinosaurs in it. His job was to dig and find them. Other children loved that exercise; not Andrew. The nerve endings on his fingers were so damaged that any contact was painful. It hurt even for Scott to rub lotion on them. To Andrew the rice felt like little knife edges. The therapists found his reactions similar to those of a severe burn victim.

Soon Andrew found a way to compensate. He would lift items by pinching them between his knuckles. Rebecca considered it a clever way to avoid using his fingertips, but the therapists felt differently. If he didn't do exercises the right way, he would not progress. Both Casey and Lori had experience with contractures. They knew kids who, after years, couldn't color a picture or throw a ball. So they would not let Andrew off easy. He began to get resistant.

...

Lori and Casey knocked on the door at their usual mid-morning time.

"We're here." Today, they said, we're going to—

"No." Andrew cut them off. He wasn't interested.

They set up anyway. Ready to start, Andrew?

"I have to go to the bathroom." Rebecca remembered him pulling the same trick at church. Sometimes he had to go three or four times, depending on how long the priest talked.

Casey and Lori ended up writing *NA* on his chart: Not Available. They had to do this often. Sometimes it meant he was in the midst of a medical procedure. Other times Andrew dozed through their morning appointment, having stayed up too late. Lori wondered if he did so on purpose. There were a lot of NA's. They often had to come back six or seven times a day to make sure they got in a session with him.

The Batesons sat down again with Dr. D'Amato. The main goal, he said, was to get Andrew walking on his prosthetics.

Rebecca thought, *Get him walking? He can't even sit.*

Scott asked if Andrew would be able to run again.

D'Amato didn't know.

Scott chose not to push him for more specifics, such as riding a bicycle. What was Dr. D'Amato supposed to say?

Scott asked the therapists if they could leave the small dinosaurs in the room. On his own, Scott tried coaxing Andrew to pick them up. He wasn't having much success. It was the same with other items. It left Andrew frustrated.

"Mommy," Andrew said, "am I ever going to hold a cup again?"

"Honey," she said, "someday you will."

"I'll be able to do stuff like Erin?"

"Mom and Dad feel someday you'll be able to do everything you could before." Rebecca realized she was overpromising, but it was hard not to.

. . .

Scott remembered the tape some friends had brought about a child with prosthetic legs. The Batesons had put it aside, neither being ready to face it, but now, while Andrew was sleeping, Scott put it in the VCR. It was evening. Scott had a nervous, butterfly feeling. He didn't really want to see it, but at the same time he did. The tape started to play. It showed a little boy riding a bicycle. The boy was wearing shorts. He was doing pretty good, but all Scott could focus on were those two prosthetic legs. It was a slap of reality. Here was Andrew's future. Scott watched it until the end. He couldn't shake that feeling of sadness.

When Rebecca came into the room, Scott told her she might want to take a look. He pushed the Play button. Watching it a second time left him with mixed thoughts. It was good to see such a child active, but how Andrew would get to that point Scott didn't have the slightest idea. The boy in the video was clearly exceptional. That wouldn't be every kid. The two watched the tape quietly. When it was over they didn't say much to each other. Andrew continued sleeping.

Mrs. Pinksaw, Andrew's kindergarten teacher, was reading to him when the nurses came in to change his dressings. His wounds had a long way to go. Mrs. Pinksaw got up to leave, but the Batesons asked if she would stay. Mrs. Pinksaw continued reading. It was real hard for her; she could see big, angry sores, including one on Andrew's upper left arm that went to the muscle. At one point Andrew was laughing at the story, then Mrs. Pinksaw caught a little scream and saw the look on his face. Still, the nurses said it was one of the easier times they had with dressings. Mrs. Pinksaw kept at it. You do what you have to do.

Casey and Lori decided to try therapy in the hospital rehab gym. They sat Andrew on a floor mat. Lori knelt behind him, Casey in front, bracing his upper body with their hands. The test was whether he could sit upright on his own. They doubted it, since he couldn't even hold up his head, but they had to start somewhere.

"Okay, Andrew," Lori said. "You be really strong, because we're going to let go." As soon as they did, Andrew slumped to one side. They kept at it, catching him before he went over. He had to rest every few minutes, which involved lying him all the way down. Rebecca thought it was like watching someone who was paralyzed. At other times, it reminded her of when he was an infant. It was almost the same process.

Slowly, Andrew learned to sit. The next goal was to have him reach to each side without toppling. He couldn't. Over he'd go. He had no trunk strength. Scott noted that his coordination was gone, too.

The therapists came up with an idea. Instead of having him lean, Casey and Lori gave him a little shove. Andrew didn't seem to mind that. He did slightly better when it was a matter of fighting back. Rebecca found this exercise hard to watch.

On August 20, about three weeks after waking up, Andrew said he wanted to see his legs. Rebecca hesitated, so it wasn't done. Lori thought: *Andrew was ready, but his mother wasn't.* Still, Lori considered it an important moment. Andrew was facing things.

Scott found himself thinking more about the future. He wondered how this might change Andrew. He had always been up for every activity: baseball, soccer, and, each fall, a swimming program at Providence College. Scott knew plenty of kids who didn't want the hassle of a pool on certain days. But Andrew was always game. That ran through Scott's mind now. Would Andrew be able to swim again? Would he think he couldn't? Maybe be too embarrassed about his legs to try? Scott assumed so. He'd probably wear long pants only and hold back from things. As he sat in Andrew's room, all those thoughts ran through Scott's mind.

The Batesons thought it time to let Andrew's friends visit. He wasn't looking great, but he was talking more. He was also in a wheelchair, so if they wanted to, everyone could go for a walk. Scott wasn't sure what the reaction would be. Some adults had seemed afraid of coming into the room, and he assumed it would be even scarier for kids.

As it turned out, children were different. They rushed in happily and just said, "Hi, Andrew. How you doing?" They studied how his pajamas covered his legs but didn't make a big deal out of it. They were mostly just curious. There was none of the hand-wringing concern you saw with certain grown-ups.

When Andrew's friends visited, the Batesons left the room so the children could talk about whatever children talk about. Sometimes Scott would peek in. Two or three kids would be sitting on the bed around some gift-wrapped toy, saying, "Let's open it—hey, cool, what's it do?" Kid stuff, first-grade stuff. Andrew was still pretty wiped, but it was a nice picture, seeing him with his buddies again.

During one such visit everyone decided to go down to the hospital garden, which had playground equipment. Scott lowered Andrew's legs into one of those swings designed for little kids. As usual, he had on long pajamas. Some of Andrew's friends helped push, but, being kids, they soon ran to other stuff. That was fine; Scott couldn't expect them to hover every second. Then he noticed a look on Andrew's face as if he was thinking, *I'm here, and can't go there.*

"Andrew," Scott said, "what's the matter, bud?"

"Nothing."

Scott put him back in the wheelchair, and the friends pushed him around. Then they went to explore again while Andrew watched.

It got to be dusk. "Andrew, you tired, buddy?"

"Yeah, I want to go upstairs."

"Your friends are still here," said Scott.

"I want to go upstairs, Dad."

They settled him back in bed. It left Scott dejected; he pictured Andrew stuck in a wheelchair, watching everyone else have fun. If that was how this played out, well . . . it worried him.

Later, Rebecca asked Scott if he had noticed Andrew's mood.

"Yeah. He looked real sad."

She thought out loud, wondering what Andrew's life would be like.

"I don't know. I don't know, Rebecca."

It wasn't something Scott was able to talk about.

The physical therapists had a soft spot for Andrew—for all the Batesons, really. They seemed such a perfect little family, then everything was just ripped up. At the same time, Andrew could be exasperating. He was quite the manipulator.

Casey Little told Andrew they had to straighten each finger five times for a count of ten. Because of the contractures, it was a painful exercise.

Ready?

How about two times? Andrew said.

Casey offered a compromise: Four.

No, Andrew said, one. He didn't play by the rules of negotiation.

"Three is my last offer," Casey said.

Fine, three.

She knew three was too few, so she drew each stretch out.

"Eight, nine, nine and a quarter, nine and a half . . ."

Andrew had a good enough sense of humor to think that was funny. But not every session. Sometimes he'd cry. It was a painful cry, with real tears. He hated that exercise.

Casey made hand-splints for Andrew to wear while he slept. That way they could hold a stretch for hours.

When the time came, Andrew always put up a fight. Scott stepped up to the job of making him put them on. Rebecca didn't have it in her.

"Do I have to wear those again?" Andrew would say.

"Yeah you do, Andrew," Scott said. "You do. I know it really rots right now. But it's going to make your hands and your fingers better." Then he thought: *Right, try to tell that to a six-year-old.*

They advised Scott first to soak his son's hands in warm water to relax them, but Andrew cried anyway. He hated the splints. Scott felt bad about having to push it. A few times Andrew wore him down so much that Scott gave in. But he usually held the line. It made him feel like the bad guy.

Andrew's favorite subject, even more than sports, was Harley-Davidson motorcycles. That's what he told Casey and Lori. Actually, he told just about everybody. One day, outside the hospital, Rebecca heard a pack of loud mufflers, or whatever it was on motorcycles that made noise. John Lamberton, Scott's brother-in-law, looked out the window to see fifty or so bikes swarming the entrance circle. Friends of friends had mentioned Andrew to a Harley person, who organized it. A number of riders came marching up to visit him. They were burly biker people, walking down the hall in a kind of gang. Some had biker-type beards. One or two seemed seven feet tall. They brought Andrew some Harley patches and a skull bandanna. Then they made him an honorary member of their Harley organization. The noise of mufflers filled the hospital as they roared away.

Joe Mullen from across the street knew that Andrew had always been a Harley type of kid. Put it this way: Joe never heard him talk about Suzukis or Kawasakis.

"You're not going to have a motorcycle," Rebecca would tell Andrew. "Not while I'm around. Not in my house." Joe Mullen didn't say anything, but he had a guess how it would turn out. When a boy talks about Harleys the way Andrew did, he's going to have a motorcycle.

Neither Mullen nor his wife had ever been to a Harley store, but they figured that was the place to get something for Andrew. They found a good one near Providence. It had plenty to choose from. They picked some cheap items, then saw a tiny black leather jacket. It cost $159. Joe, a painter, never spent $159 on something he didn't need. Out of the question. But this was an easy call. He counted out the money. He didn't consider it a big sacrifice. It was nothing, not a thing, and it was worth every dime the moment they saw Andrew put it on.

Lori LaFrance considered it quite funny. Often, the therapists found Andrew in bed wearing not just the jacket, but shades and a skull bandanna. Underneath it all there'd be this big grin. His Harley getup just put him in a good mood.

Andrew told people that *Grease* was his favorite movie. When Lori asked why, he said that everyone in it wore black leather jackets. Robin Vargas, the social worker, nicknamed him Zuko, after Danny Zuko, the movie's lead. It caught on. When Andrew was wheeled into a room wearing the jacket, everyone said, "Zuko's here." He usually had the shades on, too. They'd wheel him around the hospital that way. Andrew enjoyed the attention. That alter-ego personality was a good coping mechanism for him.

Although Andrew was at last able to keep food down, there was now another eating issue: He only ate what he wasn't supposed to. Casey often saw him push away a normal meal and later go through a whole bag of potato chips, or a box of Warheads, his favorite candy. She saw it as a control thing.

Rebecca enabled him, and admitted as much. Nothing, Rebecca thought, lowered a mother's standards like a child who wouldn't eat. She began offering Andrew Skittles and ice cream for lunch. She no longer cared whether it was good for him, as long as he kept it down. They still had the nasogastric tube in just in case, and Rebecca would do anything to keep from going back to it.

Casey Little realized that for Andrew it wasn't just about having junk, but sneaking it. At one point she saw Andrew refuse a milk shake from his mother. Shortly afterward, when Rebecca had left the room, Casey peeked in. Andrew was drinking the shake. Obviously, it was a defiance thing. He was a strong-willed child.

. . .

Lori and Casey wheeled Andrew to the sixth-floor whirlpool room. Inside were two stainless-steel bathtubs. Andrew now needed water agitation to remove dead skin. It was the same procedure given acute burn victims. Both parents had come along. As the therapists started to unwrap the outer dressing, the Batesons held up a sheet to block any view of Andrew's legs. He was back to not wanting to look. So far the parents hadn't looked either.

They got the dressings down to the final two-by-two pads underneath. This was the hard part. The pads often stuck.

As soon as any little thing hurt, Andrew shouted for them to stop. Don't pull, he said. Wait. Pretty soon Andrew was in a regular two-year-old tantrum. Lori poured sterile water on the most adhered bandages to loosen them. That calmed him, but only briefly.

"Andrew," said Lori, "we have to do this." This wasn't her favorite part of the job.

He asked for a break, just five more minutes.

Casey and Lori hoped the parents would help move it along, but they tended to do the opposite. Especially Rebecca. "Okay, hon," she said. "We'll stop."

Casey Little realized she might have behaved the same way had this been her child, but it sure dragged the process out.

The parents held up the sheet as Casey and Lori lifted Andrew into the agitation tub. The more stubborn squares needed to be submerged in moving water to be loosened. After a few minutes, several came off, but others held fast to his skin, and those Lori had to pull. That started the battle again.

Don't, Andrew would say. Wait.

Lori noticed that he yelled even when she wasn't pulling. He really did like running the show. Finally, they got the last of the pads off. Andrew had to remain in the water thirty minutes more while the agitation cleaned the wounds. All the while, Lori and Casey used sponges to rub off more dead skin. Sometimes they needed to remove small pieces with tweezers and scissors. They had to be quite thorough, dead tissue being an ideal medium for bacteria. It was a tough process.

The one trick that worked was to get Andrew talking on a subject he liked. Once he was resisting the whirlpool when Casey turned to Lori: "Did you see that Harley outside this morning?" Andrew started to ask about it. The moment the discussion was over, though, he began resisting again. On the worst days he complained so much of pain they had to give him morphine. Going to such a step, thought Lori, was more typical of a toddler who had no ability to reason, which was where Andrew was sometimes.

The parents kept the sheet drawn over the tub, and, afterward, held it up as they lifted him out. Lori and Casey would have preferred they let Andrew look. Part of their job was to get him to accept his situation. He needed to grow comfortable with his new appearance. But the parents wanted to protect him.

After the whirlpool, Casey and Lori laid Andrew down on a cushioned table covered with sterile cloths. The wound on his upper left arm was almost to the bone. They cleaned it a final time with a Q-tip, then packed it with damp gauze. There was another big lesion on his hip. The therapists could remember few other meningococcemia patients with wounds as severe.

The heat in the room was kept high so Andrew wouldn't get cold. Casey and Lori wore full precautions. By the time the session was over, Lori's clothing and hair were damp. She could feel the sweat dripping off her. It was some ordeal. Each session should have taken an hour but usually stretched to two. They had to do this twice a day.

In mid-August, Scott went back to work at the printing company. The transition was difficult. He had spent the last six weeks in the hospital. It was especially hard to be away from Andrew. He called the room every few hours.

. . .

Casey wheeled Andrew up to a table in the fine-motor room. It was late August.

The exercise was to pick up pennies by pinching them between his thumb and forefinger. Andrew used his pinkie and ring finger.

"Come on, Andrew," Casey said, but he kept doing it his way. Casey offered a deal. How about if they alternated? Every other one had to be a good pinch. With Andrew she was always making deals.

"I need to go to the bathroom."

Can't it wait?

"I need to really bad."

Rebecca took him. Usually it wasn't as immediate as he made it sound. The therapists were impressed with how creatively Andrew got out of things. When Casey acted stern, he would do something silly, like imitate Lori's southern accent to make her laugh. When whining didn't save him, he switched tactics.

"I don't love you anymore," he said.

Con men, thought Lori, *could take lessons from this child.*

Andrew was especially resistant when Mom was there. She usually took his side. One morning he wouldn't get out of bed to go to therapy; he flat-out refused. It was a standoff. Finally, Casey and Lori began to offer a compromise. Andrew could have therapy in his room today, but had to promise to go to the gym tomorrow, and—

"Okay," Rebecca said to Andrew, "you can do it tomorrow." She went for deals faster than he did. Lori and Casey thought she wasn't doing Andrew any favors.

The therapists saw this often with handicapped kids. Moms and dads grew lenient with them. Sometimes that caused problems in a family. Siblings got resentful, and the indulged child ended up ruling the roost. It was happening here. Andrew controlled things; he had his parents trained.

. . .

Once Casey and Lori took Andrew for a whirlpool session without either parent. They were able to finish in an hour instead of two. He barely acted out at all. He seemed to know the therapists weren't about to give him slack on their own. When only Scott came, it was also an improvement. Lori said to Casey, "He's got Mom's number." Andrew seemed to know this himself, and would ask Mom to come to therapy. He knew she would let him get away with a lot.

Andrew was in the whirlpool when he again said he wanted to take a peek at his legs. This time Rebecca went along with it. The two took a quick glance under the sheet. Rebecca tried not to look shocked, but her heart broke. There it was—there was the reality. It didn't seem to hit Andrew that badly. His reaction was more like curiosity from a boy's point of view. He was checking it out. A few times the sheet got caught in the whirlpool and dragged free. The two of them didn't look away. It began to get less scary.

Over time, Casey thought the parents got more on their side. Scott and Rebecca started using a reward system to get Andrew to cooperate. If he did his therapy, he would get to buy something at the gift shop. Maybe bribery wasn't ideal parenting, Rebecca thought, but it worked.

They drew up posters with therapy goals for the day: twenty quad sets, each leg. Hand stretching with Dad, twenty minutes. Wear hand-splints all night. Sit up in the wheelchair for two hours. The posters helped; Andrew liked a challenge, though it never hurt to throw in the gift shop.

Andrew liked teasing the therapists. He made a joke about Casey Little's last name by calling her Tiny. He also called her Red, that being her hair color. He played with Lori LaFrance's southern accent. She was from Georgia. He would repeat what she said, but with heavier emphasis, rolling out a lot of "Hey, y'alls."

Lori often told him, "Andrew, if you don't straighten up, I'll give you a whuppin' with my bag of switches." Andrew liked that expression, and began using it with other kids in the rehab room, warning that he would give them a whupping with Lori's bag of switches. He meant it jokingly, but not all took it that way, and Lori realized she had to be careful. You never knew what would come back out of Andrew's mouth.

Two of the therapists were named Kristen. Andrew referred to Kristen Montgomery as Big Kristen, since, at five foot six, she was five inches taller than the other Kristen. She laughed, but told Andrew it wasn't always polite to use the word *big* to describe ladies. After that, he used it constantly.

Sometimes, if Mary St. Jacques had a moment, she left the emergency room for the fifth floor to see how Andrew was doing. She was amused by the way he manipulated everyone. He was smart as a whip, and had this cute little smile. She felt there was some spirit getting back into him.

He once brought in a whoopee cushion. The therapists figured it out soon enough, but everyone took a turn being an unsuspecting victim, which really did it for Andrew. That was his idea of humor.

After therapy one day, Scott wheeled Andrew outside for a walk. He liked it, and it became a kind of routine.

Dr. Kleinman often noticed the Batesons pushing Andrew outdoors in his wheelchair. His sister, Erin, was usually with them, and, often, so were friends. To Kleinman, that was always a nice picture: Andrew and his buddies.

Still, the therapists saw Andrew as kind of a Jekyll and Hyde. He was agreeable when "off-duty," but a handful otherwise. Toward the end of August, the fifth-floor case manager wrote in his chart, "Andrew has been acting out and becoming increasingly uncooperative in both his therapy and general care." It got Casey and Lori thinking. Perhaps it was his way of saying he wanted to go home. They suggested it at the next meeting of Andrew's team. It was earlier than the doctors had planned, but they agreed it was time. They scheduled Andrew's discharge for August 30.

The evening before, Rebecca went home to College Road to get things ready. It was her first time on the block in eight weeks. Neighbors had kept up the house for her, but she cleaned anyway. She went especially heavy on the disinfectant. As she scrubbed things, she felt as upbeat as she had since this started.

Cindy Day was across the street in her home when the doorbell rang. It was Rebecca. Cindy knew she was back, having gone over a few times to help. From the kitchen, Cindy called for Rebecca to come in. Rebecca asked if Cindy could come out. It was 8 P.M. Cindy told the kids to put on their pajamas.

The two women sat outside on the stairs. "I just got a phone call from Scott," Rebecca said. "Andrew's not coming home." They had found a bone infection in his arm. It was from one of the deeper lesions. They needed to operate to clean it up. It would push things back a week.

Rebecca asked: "When is God going to decide we've had enough?"

Cindy got each of them a glass of wine. "You've come this far," she said. "Don't lose sight of the end. It's just a little setback."

Then Cindy's kids came out, and it was Mom-this, and Mom-that. Rebecca apologized for taking Cindy away from her family at bedtime.

"They're fine," Cindy said, and sent the kids back up. That was when Rebecca began to cry. Cindy had only seen her fall apart a few times all summer. As they sat together, Cindy's heart really ached for Rebecca. She had been so looking forward to getting back to their lives.

They rescheduled Andrew's homecoming for September 6, the Friday of Labor Day weekend. Maria Amaral was having coffee in the hospital garden with Rebecca. The bone infection was improving, and the staff saw no more delays, but Rebecca seemed low.

"You don't look well," Maria said.

Rebecca explained that Andrew had been asking a lot of questions about the future. She hadn't been up to answering, feeling like she would cry if she tried. Maria had seen some of those moments. Scott had jumped in and handled it.

"I think I'm losing it," said Rebecca.

Perhaps, Maria thought, some of it had to do with a change in Scott. He seemed stronger. Maybe Rebecca was able to let her guard down now that Scott was there to hold the fort.

"You did it long enough," said Maria. "Now it's his turn."

Rebecca didn't say anything for a moment. Then: "I wish I could jump over that fence and keep running." Maria just put her arm around her. Sometimes, she said, problems do become too much. It was normal to want to escape.

Karen Zelano saw the change in Scott too. Early on, Rebecca was strong for both of them. Now the two seemed to switch roles, Rebecca acting the more emotional. Over the next days, Maria kept expecting Rebecca to really fall apart, but she didn't. Maybe Rebecca was afraid to let it happen. Maria never figured that one out.

Scott knew he'd had a lot of low moments back in the PICU. Rebecca seemed to be having some of her own now. Scott didn't go there, though. He didn't want to get into a discussion about whose turn it was to feel lower. He felt that would just make the whole thing weaker.

It made Rebecca feel more alone than ever.

On September 4, a few days before going home, Andrew was due to be fitted for his new legs. That morning he was more uncooperative than usual. Lori found it a surprise, this being such an upbeat step. He was lying on a floor mat, with Rebecca nearby. They were preparing to cast him for the prosthetics, but Andrew wanted no part of it. He began to resist to the point of yelling. He beat the mat with his arms. He was beyond the point where you could reason with him. Lori had never seen him this bad. He turned most of it on Rebecca.

"I hate you, Mom," he yelled. He must have repeated it fifteen times. He put his face in one of his hands and kept thrashing. It got so bad that later one of the doctors decided to order him a sedative. Perhaps, Casey thought, being fitted for new legs got Andrew facing what had happened to him. There was no particular reason for him to turn against Rebecca, except that in Lori's experience, moms always got it the worst.

Chapter 12

"We just have to keep doing it, pal . . ."

Rebecca left Providence at 7 A.M. with her sister Deb. They planned to look at four facilities, from Rhode Island to Boston.

Andrew's team had recommended that Scott and Rebecca find him a sleep-in rehabilitation hospital. He would need two months of six-hour-a-day therapy. Hasbro Children's offered outpatients only a few sessions a week.

Rebecca hated the idea. Another hospital? She needed to get some normalcy in their lives. Plus, she wanted to sleep on something that wasn't vinyl. The Hasbro team understood, but thought he belonged in a round-the-clock facility. Learning to walk as a bilateral amputee was a considerable challenge, to say nothing of Andrew's hands. The only logical choice was in-residence rehab.

All right. Rebecca would see what was out there. She would try it their way.

Rebecca and Deb arrived at their first stop. It was in a strip plaza.

Rebecca asked if they had a tilt-table.

No.

Parallel bars?

No.

Don't you need those to teach Andrew to walk?

Well, they could try a harness.

Rebecca didn't want them improvising on her son, looking it up in some book and saying, "We'll experiment with this."

The next two stops had the feel of geriatric centers. That wasn't what Rebecca had in mind either. Nor did they have broad experience with Andrew's situation. She was learning that child bilateral amputees were not a common occurrence.

Close to 6 P.M., she arrived at their last stop, in Boston, an hour's drive from home. The facility focused more on head traumas than limb loss, but it was geared to kids. It was the only place remotely close to what Rebecca was looking for.

She asked the director if she could bring Andrew as an outpatient.

Given Andrew's needs, he said, full-time would be best. It would even cost the family less. Insurance covered 100 percent of inpatient rehabilitation, but only 80 percent of outpatient. That didn't make sense to Rebecca, since inpatient was more expensive, but those were the rules.

She worked out the math in her head. For outpatient they'd have to pay $500 or so in cash per week. She wasn't sure how they could afford that. But neither could she make her son sleep in another hospital for two months. They'd commute. Outpatient was the only choice. She'd find a way, take on debt; it would be worth it.

Money issues aside, the director felt strongly that Andrew needed to be an inpatient.

At that Rebecca broke down. "I need to go home at night," she said. "I have a daughter. I have a husband. We have to get back to living." Maybe, she said, Andrew would get better physically as an inpatient, but not emotionally. She couldn't stop sobbing.

The director relented. If she could afford to pay, he would work it out.

All right, Rebecca said, she and Andrew would come as outpatients.

. . .

As they drove back to Hasbro, Deb asked Rebecca if she was sure. Commuting to Boston, known for road congestion, would be a nightmare.

Rebecca said she'd tough it out. She would drop Erin at school before nine o'clock, drive Andrew to Boston for a ten-thirty start, stay until four, then drive home.

"You're going to do this twice a day in rush-hour traffic?" said Deb. It could be ninety minutes or more each way. "Are you sure you're making the right decision?"

Down deep, Rebecca wasn't. It would be exhausting. It might not give Andrew all he needed. But she could not check into another hospital.

"Yes, I'm sure."

They got back to Hasbro at 8 P.M. Rebecca told Scott her decision. By the next morning, she was a mess. Maybe she should choose inpatient. No, she couldn't do that to Andrew. Then again, was it right to make him sit in a car three hours a day? There were no good choices. She had to make a decision, and outpatient was it.

Andrew's rehab team knew about Rebecca's dilemma. Although they had recommended a sleep-in facility, most felt torn about it. At their next meeting they talked about another option. Could they themselves handle Andrew as a full-time outpatient? It would be a first. Hasbro was only staffed to give outpatients an hour or two a week. Andrew would need five to six hours a day. They couldn't shortchange others, so it would mean long shifts for months. It was a stressful meeting.

Late in the afternoon, the therapists sat down with the Batesons and asked about their plans for Andrew. Rebecca explained that she couldn't face another hospital, so she had worked out a commuter schedule with the Boston rehab center. She dreaded the driving and the cost, but felt it was her only option.

Casey Little asked if Rebecca might be open to another choice.

Which?

"We had a meeting," said Casey, "and we've all agreed to treat Andrew on a full outpatient basis here."

But Rebecca thought they weren't geared for such intense therapy.

Casey explained they had gotten involved with Andrew. They wanted to see him through this.

It was one big weight off her shoulders.

About eight staffers were at the exit meeting at the hospital, including a woman from United HealthCare, the Batesons' insurance company. She told Rebecca the firm had decided to cover Andrew's outpatient therapy 100 percent. It was a tremendous relief. Rebecca had begun worrying about how they would keep their house.

The mayor of Providence, Buddy Cianci, had been at the church fund-raiser, and promised that Andrew would come home in a city fire truck with police escort. Joe Mullen watched from across the street as the kids decorated the block with streamers. The idea was for the fire truck to drive through them, like a finish line. Everyone began cheering when they heard the police sirens. It was around 2 P.M., September 9, 1997. Andrew sat by Scott on the front seat of the truck. Joe Mullen thought: *Jeepers crow, never seen anything like it.*

The first thing Andrew wanted to do was see his room. It had been sixty-seven days. Scott carried him up. Back downstairs, Scott put him in his wheelchair and his friends pushed him this way and that. The next thing Andrew wanted to do was ride his bike, or at least sit on it. It was the one that looked like a Harley. Scott lugged it from the basement, braced Andrew on the seat, and walked him up and down the sidewalk.

"Dad," Andrew said, "I hope I can ride again."

For Scott it was a bittersweet moment. Andrew still looked sick. There were deep circles under his eyes. He still had the nasogastric tube in his nose.

. . .

Rebecca didn't think about sleeping arrangements until later that night. The Batesons lived in a small, two-story cape, with Scott and Rebecca's bedroom downstairs and the kids up. They felt Andrew should not be on a different floor. Besides, Andrew's room had a single bed at bunk height. Rebecca wasn't comfortable with that.

They put him on the pull-out couch in the living room. Erin didn't want to be alone upstairs, so she slept on the couch too. There was only one bathroom in the house, on the first floor. The stairs, Rebecca realized, were going to be a problem.

Every time they thought they had things figured out, something else came up. Andrew, unable to sit upright for more than thirty seconds or so, was nervous about taking a bath. Rebecca called ambulatory care stores to see if they carried a bath seat. They did. Rebecca was relieved until they told her the cost. Instead, she got a beach chair from the basement, cleaned it with soap and water, then bleached it. She did the same to the bathtub. Andrew still had open wounds, and she worried about infection. She put a towel down on the tub floor, the beach chair on the towel, and sat Andrew down like that. When they were done, Rebecca scooped him up and out. Afterward, she was as wet as he. Being home was a relief, but it was also a hassle.

There were a lot of home-care supplies that Rebecca had to order. United HealthCare never questioned her. So far, the policy had covered everything 100 percent—the whole hospitalization. There hadn't been a single "Why are you having an MRI instead of a CAT scan?" Rebecca knew that many people had health-insurance frustrations, but in her own case, she wasn't seeing that.

Rebecca and Andrew left College Road for therapy at Hasbro. On the way, he asked if this was the route they took the morning they went to the emergency room.

"Yes."

Was this how fast they went?

"No. Mommy and Daddy were going faster."

Andrew seemed fixated on that. He wanted to know just how quickly they had gotten him there. He asked about it every day.

The closer they got to the hospital, the more Andrew's voice tensed. Usually, by the time they pulled into the parking lot, he felt ill. Rebecca was glad she always kept a bowl in the car.

Within a few days, Andrew became as stubborn as before he was discharged. Casey told him to pick up a penny and hold it five seconds. He picked it up for one.

"Andrew . . ."

He did it for a second and a half.

"Come on, Andrew."

He picked it up. Casey began to count. "One . . . two . . . thr—"

He dropped it.

She knew it was hard for him, but he was also testing her.

"Okay, Andrew, we'll get back to that. Let's move on."

The therapists put a vest on him with oversized buttons. Andrew's job was to fasten them with thumb and forefinger. He couldn't. They tried putting the buttons halfway through. Andrew still cheated, finishing them with his ring finger and pinky. He had trouble with a zipper vest, too. He couldn't get a grip on the pull-tab; he had no hand strength. It worried Scott. These were the most basic skills, but for Andrew they were big mountains to climb.

The therapists tried burying plastic dinosaurs in putty instead of rice; Andrew would have to pull it apart. That was a tough exercise for him. His hands were still curled and painful. He continued to grip items between his knuckles. Casey was getting discouraged about how far his hands would come back. They were still supertight and sensitive from lesions.

Robin Vargas's social work office was around the corner from rehab. She sometimes heard the back and forth.

"Andrew, you have to pinch correctly."

"Just a sec . . ."

"Andrew . . ."

"Not yet . . ."

Then it would turn into negotiation.

"Five times."

"Two," Andrew would answer.

"Four."

"Okay," said Andrew, "one."

Because of his resistance, it was routine for the therapists to stay late at work, leaving around 7 P.M. For Lori LaFrance, this was one of the hardest cases of her career. Occasionally, she went back to the private office to vent.

"That kid's driving me up a wall," she said.

Casey Little understood. Andrew may have been physically frail, but mentally he could wear down any of them. Kristen Montgomery thought he was among the most impaired children she had worked with, and the most stubborn. Even so, she liked him, and respected that he had everyone's number.

Soon they began to get his number, too. They knew Andrew performed better when he had control, so they made a list of ten exercises, told him he had to do five, and let him pick three. Andrew thought he'd won a big concession. He barely noticed that the therapists got to choose the other two.

Treacy Lewander, another physical therapist, began bringing in Atomic Warheads for rewards. She had never heard of them, but Andrew said they were his favorite candy. At one point Andrew had Treacy sample one. It fizzed uncomfortably in her mouth. Andrew liked that she thought it tasted horrible. He got a kick out of things like that.

They often played a match game with cards. The goal was to make Andrew pick them up to improve his pinching ability. Instead, he dragged them to the edge of the table and flipped them.

"Andrew, you have to pick them up right."

"I am." At that point, he dragged the cards and flipped them quickly, as if no one had time to see.

Lori joined the game as his opponent and said that from now on, his matches wouldn't count unless he flipped cards the honest way. He began to do so; he was very competitive.

Anything to do with sports usually brought out a spark in Andrew. Lori gave him a light plastic basketball as he sat in the rehab room. His job was to hold it between his curled hands and shoot toward a toy basket. That forced him to work on sitting balance. He didn't resist much during that exercise.

Scott continued to stretch Andrew's fingers at home. Andrew clearly dreaded those sessions. They usually did it before bedtime.

"Dad, do we have to, Dad?"

"Andrew, I know you hate doing this, but someday you'll be glad."

"It hurts, Dad. It hurts, it hurts, it hurts."

It was tough on Scott, but he made Andrew push that stretch. Rebecca often wished Scott would give Andrew a night off. Once Scott did, but the next day Casey showed him that Andrew's hands were stiffer. That made Scott stricter about it.

"We have to, bud," Scott said. Didn't Andrew want to hold a pencil one day? Or his bike handlebars? "This is how you'll get to where you were before."

"When, Dad? When's that going to happen?"

"We just have to keep doing it, pal." It was hard to explain to a six-year-old why something that hurt so badly was good for him.

Sometimes the splint argument got Andrew asking why this whole illness happened to him. Scott never knew a good answer.

"Andrew, I don't know."

"But why, Dad?"

Scott explained that this bad disease just got inside him, and now they had to make him the best they could.

That didn't satisfy Andrew. He kept asking why. This was how Scott's nights often went.

. . .

At day's end, Rebecca told Scott that Andrew had thrown up again when they pulled into the hospital lot for therapy. She was looking for a shoulder, but the news left Scott frustrated. Last week, he said, Andrew was doing good, and now he's throwing up. Why couldn't they find what was wrong with his stomach? Scott hated hearing about setbacks. He had been high about them coming home, but that was fading. Andrew just didn't seem to be improving much. Scott's instinct was to keep asking why they couldn't solve it.

He wasn't blaming Rebecca, but it still left her feeling pushed away.

Rebecca heard Scott pull into the driveway; he was back from work. She felt a knot in her stomach. Scott came inside and hugged the children. Rebecca stood apart. Scott did not approach her. The two had never been that public with affection, but lately there was a greater distance.

Scott did not ask about her day, nor did Rebecca ask how work had gone. She knew he didn't want to waste time with small talk.

"How was therapy?" asked Scott. What had Andrew done?

She began to talk about it, which she needed to do, but Scott interrupted.

Did Rebecca feel Andrew was better? Did he improve in any way?

She felt like he was grilling her, as if it was Rebecca's fault that progress was slow.

That wasn't Scott's intention; he just wanted to know right off if Andrew had made headway. Was the problem being solved?

Rebecca said that he sat for forty-five seconds at one point. That was better than the day before. She was thrilled about it. Scott's reaction was less so.

"Shouldn't he be sitting fine by now?" he asked. "When is he going to sit by himself?"

Rebecca said the pace of therapy had been slow. Andrew had

resisted some things, so they hadn't been able to work with his fingers, and—

"Why not?" Scott asked. It was his way of expressing frustration. To Rebecca, it felt like he was blaming her.

A month or so after getting home from the hospital, the Batesons were at a big event downtown called WaterFire: thousands of people walking by fiery braziers set above the surface of the Providence River. Andrew was in his wheelchair. Various aunts, uncles, and cousins had come along; it was a big family to-do. At one point, they began up a long set of outdoor stairs. Aunt Jen carried Andrew while Rebecca and Scott took the chair. The other kids charged ahead. At that, Andrew started to sob; he was crying hard. He said he wanted his legs back. He didn't want to do this anymore.

"Where are they, Mommy?" he said. "I want to go get them."

No one knew how to react. His breakdown seemed to come out of the blue. Rebecca took him from Jen.

"Honey, they're gone."

Andrew pointed to the white, domed Rhode Island State capitol. "They're in that building," he said. "I want to go get them right now."

"Why do you think they're in there, Andrew?"

"Because Dr. D'Amato said they were in Washington."

While in the hospital, Andrew had asked the surgeon what happened to his legs. Dr. D'Amato said he had sent them to a lab in Washington to be tested. Andrew had once been shown a picture of the U.S. Capitol and thought it was the Rhode Island State House, which looked similar. That's where he assumed his legs were.

"Honey," said Rebecca, "that's not Washington. Washington has a building that looks like that but this isn't it. It's a different building."

Andrew didn't care. He just wanted to go get them. He was sobbing hard. He asked why his mother let them take his legs off.

Rebecca explained that he would have died if they hadn't.

"Why didn't you have them fix them instead?"

Rebecca began to cry too; so did her sisters. Everyone finally said good-bye and went back to their cars. That was the first time Andrew had talked this way since the night they'd told him.

Scott worried that it was the beginning of a bad period. But it passed pretty quickly.

Soon Andrew's new legs were ready. They had no cosmetic covers because adjustments had to be made. Rebecca warned Andrew that they weren't going to look so good. Except for the feet, they were metal rods. Andrew didn't notice. Once they put them on, he seemed delighted.

Scott came home from work, and there was Andrew in his wheelchair with his new legs. It was a nice sight. "Wow, Andrew," Scott said. "They look great." Still, Scott could see that Andrew wasn't about to just stand up and walk; it wasn't going to be that easy by a long shot. At the moment, Andrew couldn't put any pressure on his legs at all.

Casey and Lori helped Andrew lie back-down on a tilt-table, strapping him at the knees, waist, and chest. They fixed the bottom of his new legs on a foot plate. The idea was to raise the table slowly to get him used to standing. They hoped to get him to 45 degrees, half of vertical. It was his first weight-bearing exercise. They began at 5 degrees, then 10. They paused at 20 for two minutes. Andrew said he was scared, but they coaxed him to 30, then 40. He remained there only a minute. His knees hurt a lot. They lowered him, but he was still crying. They felt it would take him months to stand with full weight, let alone walk.

Andrew's legs were still resolving from the trauma. At times they would swell, and then the swelling would go down. With each change, Casey and Lori had to adjust his prosthetics. They did so by changing the socks and silicone cover on his knees. They had to get the thickness just right. It was an ordeal.

. . .

They put Andrew on the tilt-table twice a day. He complained so much they couldn't leave him bearing weight as long as they needed to.

Then they had an idea. After getting him semi-upright, they put a toy basketball hoop in front of him and gave him a ball to shoot. That kept him on the table the longest of all. Kristen thought he had a good shot, especially for a kid who had to squeeze the ball between curled hands.

The technique speeded his progress. In only a week they worked him up to 80 degrees. Even Casey and Lori hadn't expected that.

They moved to the parallel bars. Andrew's arms and hands couldn't bear weight, so they needed to triple-team him. Kristen supported his hips, another therapist his knees, and a third was ready to catch him from behind. He kept buckling whenever they let go. They kept at it, though, and after several days Andrew was able to hold himself upright briefly. It was an emotional moment for everyone even though it only lasted a few seconds.

Mom kept asking when Andrew would walk on his own. No one could say, since they'd never had a bilateral amputee. Put it this way, they told Rebecca: walking was not around the corner.

"When do you think?" she asked.

You mean a step or two?

Right, a step or two.

They hoped Halloween, but maybe not. Halloween was six weeks away. Most felt they shouldn't have picked a date like that. If it didn't happen, the family would be discouraged.

Rebecca tried to tell Scott about Andrew's day. It hadn't gone well, and Rebecca was down about it. Andrew had been unable to fasten oversized buttons in therapy. She said it was hard to see him struggle like that. Rebecca was trying to keep from crying.

Scott could tell she wanted him to hold her. He couldn't bring himself to do it, though. If he did, he would probably break down too. That would turn one tear into ten minutes of tears, and he didn't think it would help for both of them to be weak. Rebecca would have seen it as a sign of strength had Scott held her, but that didn't occur to him.

Whenever Scott himself was about to break down he wanted to be alone, or for someone to change the subject. He figured Rebecca was the same.

Rebecca showed a different front to Andrew. She felt it important that they act upbeat around him. Around Erin, too. Sometimes she worried that Scott wasn't as careful; he wouldn't always hide his low moods from the children. Rebecca never found the right moment to say that, though.

Earlier, Rebecca had told herself that once Andrew got off the feeding tube, Scott would get past his anger. But he didn't.

Around then, they decided to get a new car. Rebecca thought that in its own way, this could be a turning point for Scott. It wasn't.

Maybe, she told herself, Scott would change once he planted those new bushes. Or got that component for his computer. She was grasping at anything.

Rebecca was driving home from therapy with Andrew when she saw a poster on the door of a nearby hairdresser. It was December of 1997. PLEASE HELP THE BATESONS, it said. It brought her up short. Rebecca had never seen herself as a person in that kind of need. But she knew they were not in a position to be too proud. Altogether, they had received about $40,000 from fund-raisers, which they put in a trust. They figured Andrew would need his own bathroom as a teen. That was what they would likely use it for, since their home only had one.

The therapists had Andrew stand in front of a regular table, leaning against it on his hands. Every so often he started to topple over, but they were right there to catch him. After enough of those, Andrew trusted them, which had its downside, since he needed to know there wouldn't always be somebody there.

Next, they told him to let go of the table altogether, try to stand with no handhold. He could do it only for a moment. Then they had an idea. They bet him there was no way he could stand for five seconds. At that point, he did it for ten. Telling Andrew he couldn't do something was a great motivator.

They tried to get him to weight-shift, lean on one prosthetic leg or the other. He said it hurt too much. Then Lori and Casey told Andrew to try stepping on their toes. He liked that idea. Kristen guessed it was payback. Whether he knew it or not, the game got him shifting weight.

Andrew told the therapists it was their turn to step on his own toes. When they complied, he shrugged and said, "Doesn't hurt."

Later, Andrew thought of another positive thing about his new legs. He told Casey and Lori he could go skiing and his feet wouldn't get cold. They all laughed hard over that one; they liked that he was finding the silver lining. To go from not wanting to look at his legs to saying his toes won't get cold was big.

Andrew still resisted leaning, which was necessary if he were eventually to walk. They came up with the thought of giving him a plastic bat to swing. They had to wedge it into his curled hands, but he liked the idea so much he didn't complain about pain. They put a Wiffle ball on a big tee in front of him. Treacey Lewander knelt below Andrew's belt level to brace him as he swung. She was known for trying spirited approaches. Dicey ones, too, to be honest. If she didn't stay low, those swings came close to her head.

Soon they started pitching to him. Andrew connected with some good ones; people across the small rehab gym had to duck. Usually they retreated to safer rooms. It bothered Andrew's hands, but he just shook them and tried again. At first Scott pitched, but he wasn't getting them over. A few times he hit Andrew, so Lori and Casey sent him back to the bullpen. Mom pitched next. Even she did better than Scott, which no one could figure out, since he had been a Little League coach. Sometimes Andrew hit the far office wall—a home run. He couldn't get enough of that game. There was something about hitting Wiffle balls indoors that appealed to him. Gripping that bat began to desensitize his hands.

Andrew stood between the parallel bars. One therapist held his hips, another his knees, and a third his torso. They moved a foot forward, then stopped.

Ready for another step, Andrew?

No. It hurt.

Come on, here we go.

A second step, stop.

Andrew said he had to quit.

Not yet, Andrew. Ready again?

Step . . . stop.

They made this into a regular exercise. Rebecca watched as they triple-teamed him, wondering how he would ever do this on his own.

Chapter 13

"Andrew, slow down . . ."

Andrew was sitting on the couch at home.
"Hey, Dad," he said. Then he slowly stood. He sat back down soon enough, but that was big, standing up from a sitting position with no support. It was interesting how this happened, Scott thought. Andrew spent most of his days resisting exercises at Hasbro, then made a breakthrough at home. Maybe, thought Scott, it was because it was Andrew's idea.

In October, the new owners of Scott's printing firm decided to close down their Rhode Island operation. Most employees, including Scott, lost their jobs. Many of his friends worried that it would push Scott to a breaking point. It seemed a bad blow on top of everything else. It really wasn't. To Scott there were bigger problems in this world. He had a degree in chemical technology. Perhaps he would switch to that field. Meanwhile, this allowed him to be part of Andrew's therapy again.

He and Rebecca now had to pay out of pocket to stay with United HealthCare. It more than doubled their premium to about $400 a month, but decent health insurance was a priority. The mortgage was second. After that, they'd worry about each bill as it came in.

. . .

Whenever Andrew seemed upset during rehab, it got plenty of attention from Scott and Rebecca. Maybe he was tired, the parents said, or hurting. To Casey and Lori that was no help at all. Instead of distracting Andrew from his pain, the Batesons fed into it. Nor did they have a good sense for when he was working the system. Rebecca let him get away with the most. If Andrew insisted he could only pick up three coins, not ten, Rebecca would say, "Okay, Andrew, three's fine." Occasionally, Scott told Andrew to just do it. You seldom heard that from Mom.

Once, as Andrew stood against a table, one of the therapists gave him little shoves to make him work on balance. Rebecca couldn't hold back. "Stop pushing him," she finally said. Then she apologized. She knew it had to be done.

The therapists tried telling the Batesons that physical therapy often involved tasks that appeared in parents' eyes to hurt the child. Wouldn't it be easier at such times if Scott and Rebecca left the room? Usually, the parents stayed. The therapists had seldom seen both a mom and dad so present to a child. In many cases, parents alternated, the mother by day, the father by night. Scott and Rebecca were pretty much there all the time. That was good to see. At the same time, it sure allowed Andrew to get away with things.

When other rehab kids were out of earshot Andrew was full of questions about them. Why was that one wearing that thing?

They told him it was a bone-growth device.

For what?

The child had a length discrepancy, and needed one leg bone stretched to equal the other.

How did they attach it?

The doctors drilled four pins directly into the bone.

How'd they get those pins in?

One thing Andrew knew how to do was ask questions.

Rehab had another little boy who was sort of a spitfire. He was about seven. Out of the blue he asked Andrew what happened to his legs. It was the first time anyone had done that. Kristen Montgomery, nearby, heard it. *That's all we need,* she thought. She cringed a little, worrying that Andrew would take it wrong.

Andrew froze. He looked at Lori LaFrance with a blank stare. Lori bent down to him. "You want to tell him about your boo-boos?"

Andrew was shy sometimes. "You tell him," he whispered.

"That's okay?" Lori said.

He nodded.

"Well," Lori explained, "Andrew got really sick and the doctors had to take part of his legs away. So now he's using new legs so he can learn to walk again."

At that, the other boy proudly held up his hand. "My fingers got blown off," he said. Several were indeed missing. The boy went back to what he was doing. Andrew asked Lori what happened to him. She recalled hearing that it had been a big firecracker. Lori considered it a helpful exchange. It said there was no shame in having lost something.

Andrew stood between the parallel bars. He was past the point of needing a therapist to brace him. His assignment was to try standing for a minute or more. For some reason, Kristen and Lori got a feeling, and started to look. Without saying anything, Andrew let go of the bars. Then he took a step. That wasn't supposed to have happened. At that, everyone in the room stopped. By now Andrew had grabbed hold again, but then he realized he had an audience. That seemed to do it for him. He let go and took another step, and another. Lori held her breath. Andrew turned around, took his hands off the bars, and walked back.

People began to clap. Kristen wiped away a few tears. Lori was crying too. Breakthroughs happened often enough in rehab, but for Andrew Bateson to take steps was a big one. It was late September, eight weeks after he woke from his coma. He had beaten their Halloween prediction by a good month.

The next day, Andrew's legs were sore from bearing weight, the skin by his knees inflamed. He couldn't tolerate standing or even wearing his legs; it was a big setback. The whole question of his walking outside parallel bars was put off.

Kristen wondered if this stage of therapy was too daunting for Andrew. Walking on two prosthetics, she thought, wasn't twice as hard as on one; it was ten times harder. Not having a good leg to go back to was a tough, tough problem.

Andrew showed up at Robin Vargas's door in his wheelchair. Her social-work office was around the corner from rehab. Andrew knew she had a basketball hoop inside. He wanted to know if he could practice on it. She asked what else he was doing at the moment.

"Therapy, but I want to play basketball."

A rehab person came in.

"I'm really sorry."

Robin made a suggestion. If Andrew finished what he was doing and it was okay with his therapist, could he come play later?

"I want to play now."

"Five more times," the therapist said, "and you can shoot baskets."

"Three more," Andrew said.

"Four," the therapist said.

"Two."

Robin liked to see Andrew act feisty. It was better than withdrawing. She suspected the rehab people weren't quite as thrilled by that side of him.

Andrew didn't see the point in shooting baskets if he couldn't win, so he asked Robin Vargas for a match. He went first, shooting with curled hands. He wasn't bad, but had his share of misses. The ball bounced off the rim, knocking things off her desk. Sometimes he shot wide of the hoop, sending the receiver flying off her phone.

"Sorry," he said, unconvincingly.

It was always hard to end the game.

"One more," he said.

Okay, Andrew. One more.

"And if I make this, I get another one."

Andrew often asked about Lori LaFrance's pregnancy. Her husband was a medical resident at Brown. This would be their first.

"You know whether it's a boy or a girl?"

No, Andrew.

"You gonna find out?"

Yes.

He kept asking until she had the information.

"What you going to name him?"

"William Curt Phillip LaFrance the Third." He looked at her like she was kidding. She wasn't. "Really. William Curt Phillip LaFrance the Third."

Andrew told everyone. "Lori found out her baby's going to be a boy." Then he repeated the name in his best Georgia drawl: "Weeeliumm, Kuhhht, Pheelp, Lafrayance the Thuhhhd." Lori just looked on and smiled.

Rehab had an adaptive tricycle equipped with a chest harness for children lacking trunk strength. They strapped Andrew onto it and secured his prosthetic feet to the pedals. He didn't once say he was nervous or in pain, which made everyone exchange glances. They stepped back and off he went. He circled the gym, rode into the hallway and down a long corridor. He had a little trouble holding the hand grips, but it didn't seem to hang him up.

Kristen called after him: "Andrew! You have to slow down." He didn't. Rebecca just watched, recognizing the old Andrew.

Kristen explored new bike routes with him in the hospital. The two rode the elevator to the basement, where there were tunnel-like hallways. At one point they came upon a narrow, hot corridor Kristen found creepy. "Let's hope we don't run into any rats down here," she said.

Andrew perked up at that. Rats? He tried to take off in search of them, but Kristen held on to one of the bike straps. She worried that he would run people down. Sometimes he broke away and she had to jog to catch up. A few of the basement hallways were about 100 degrees. Kristen came back to rehab sweating.

Often they wheeled past doctors, a few of whom urged him on. "Cool bike," one said. "Can I try that thing?" Jokingly, a few doctors plastered themselves against the walls as Andrew went by. At least Kristen *thought* they were joking.

Lori was with him when they came upon another long, dungeon-like corridor, this one with downhill ramps. Andrew started pedaling. Soon he was just flying. The bike was designed to be unable to flip, but Lori noticed he took some of the corners on two wheels, which she hadn't seen before. She began to think Andrew should have a helmet.

Robin Vargas occasionally saw him barreling through the lobby, a therapist chasing after him. He considered it a game to try to pedal away from them.

"Andrew," they'd be saying, "slow down. This is a crowded area."

He always had a look-at-me grin. He liked getting away with things. He only slowed if they grabbed the strap.

Sometimes he rode up to visit the nurses in PICU and on the fifth floor. Casey and Lori felt the bike was bringing his personality back. Or perhaps it was the speed factor; Andrew liked going fast. Whenever he was moving his behavior got better.

About twenty people were at the Batesons' house for Erin's ninth birthday, October 13, 1997. Andrew was sitting on a couch in the front room. Suddenly, he stood and walked across the rug to the other couch. No one helped, and he didn't hold on to anything. Andrew had just taken his first unsupported steps. That wasn't supposed to come for months. Someone said, "Did you see that?"

People crowded into the room.

Without saying anything, Andrew stood and walked back to the first couch.

Everyone started clapping. It had been three weeks since those first steps between the parallel bars. Scott got his video camera. Funny thing, he thought: here was another breakthrough at home instead of rehab. Andrew stood again and walked to the other couch.

That night it occurred to Scott that he had been excited about this same achievement when Andrew was fifteen months old. That wasn't to take away from the moment, but it was an irony.

The next day, Scott brought the videotape to rehab. He and Rebecca were ecstatic. Kristen and Lori popped it in the VCR. It was a real thrill to see Andrew walking outside parallel bars. His gait was awkward, though. If they didn't correct that, it could in time damage joints and muscles and limit progress. Kristen caught herself: There's a therapist's mentality for you, worrying about mechanics instead of celebrating a breakthrough.

On the tape, Lori noticed Erin sitting on the corner of the couch, uncharacteristically sullen. Kristen caught it too. This was Erin's birthday video, and the star was her little brother. Even now the parents didn't see it. Lori realized that Andrew may well have walked because Erin had been getting the attention. The focus hadn't been on him, and he wanted it back.

Both therapists could imagine how hard it was to be the big sister of Andrew Bateson. That had become Erin's identity. All anybody said to her was, "Erin, did you see what Andrew did today?" Most of the time, though, she handled it well. She was right there for him.

Now that he could take a few steps, Andrew didn't care about quality. When they tried to get him to work on gait, he acted like they were holding him back. It became harder than ever to talk him into fine-motor work with his hands. "Too boring," he'd say. Kristen solved this by bringing in a gun that shot little foam discs. If Andrew agreed to pick up the discs afterward with a pinch-grasp, he could shoot the therapists anywhere but the face. Scott volunteered to be shot as well. Then they noticed that Andrew had his ring finger on the trigger. They added a rule: Index finger, or no gun. That was a little tough for Andrew, given the tendon damage, but he liked shooting things enough to make the extra effort.

The prosthetic shop made him a second pair of legs for swimming. They were hollow, with a non-absorbent cover. They were designed to fill with water so they wouldn't buoy and up-end him in the small rehab pool. Andrew discovered that when he stepped out, he could make water squirt out a hole at the bottom of each leg. Robin Vargas was at the side of the pool, talking to the parents, when Andrew made one of the legs squirt in her direction. The water got on her stockings and skirt. The parents were apologetic, but it was hard for her to get angry, given how pleased it made Andrew. She decided to stop by on pool days to be a victim. Afterward, she just went back to her office and waited to dry off. It became kind of a game to both of them.

Often, Andrew's legs got sore and made him tentative, so they had to look for ways to push him those extra yards. Debbie, the rehab billing secretary, occasionally brought in treats or Beanie Babies. When Andrew said it hurt too much to walk, they told him to check if Debbie had brought anything. Somehow, he made his way to her desk.

Sports worked best. His therapists brought him to a nearby hallway to kick a soccer ball. The corridor went past the Collis Room, where the hospital's bigwigs met. Not far from the door, Kristen and Casey set up benches as goalposts. When Andrew got the ball through, they'd both yell "Goal." Even when he missed they cheered his progress.

The Collis Room's door opened. A secretary poked her head out and whispered, "There's a meeting. Could you keep it down?" She wasn't snapping at them, but she felt they should be aware that these were senior executives. As soon as she disappeared back in, Andrew whispered to Kristen and Casey, "There's a meeting—could you keep it down?"

Once, in the middle of a soccer session, the Collis Room door opened and people in suits filed out. Andrew kicked the ball right at them. It broke down their reserve. Most grinned, and one sent it right back at him. They were good sports about it. That was a relief to Casey. Still, she was struck by Andrew having little fear of these adults. Casey wouldn't have kicked a soccer ball at the hospital's executives.

They never knew what trick Treacy Lewander would use next to engage Andrew; she was known for the nuttiest ideas. One day in December they looked up to see him rolling through the gym door on a pair of Fisher-Price roller skates, Treacy holding him from behind. They had side-by-side wheels but still, Casey couldn't believe it. Roller skates on Andrew? He seemed the only one besides Treacy who didn't have a problem with it.

Later, Andrew talked Lori, who was very pregnant by now, into helping him skate. She waddled behind him, supporting him under his arms. To challenge him, she decided to let go briefly. His legs went out from under him. Lori was too slow at that stage to catch him. He went down on his back—one of his first falls with his legs on. He looked up to see how Lori would react.

"Andrew," she said, "I dropped you. You fell on the ground." Afterward, he made a point of telling everyone he wasn't going skating with Lori anymore.

It seemed to Scott that Andrew was complaining of pain less. He guessed it was because he was active again—biking, playing soccer, and such. It was now close to six months since Andrew had gotten sick.

Dr. Kleinman got a call in the PICU from Treacey Lewander. "Andrew's down here," said Treacy, "and he has something to show you."

Kleinman headed over to rehab to see what was going on. She found Andrew sitting on one of the mats with Mom. He didn't say anything when she came in. Then he stood and walked across the room. He was smiling, very pleased with himself. Dr. Kleinman gave him some applause.

"Andrew," she said, "you are amazing." She thanked them for letting her see this.

She thought back to when his family had been facing the amputations. At the time Kleinman had said to them, "He'll still be Andrew. Even without his legs." She wasn't sure they'd heard her at the time. Now she had that same thought.

Scott had been doing nightly hand-stretching with Andrew for months. The therapists were surprised that Scott had hung in there that long. To be honest, it was wearing Scott down. There hadn't been much progress.

"Dad," Andrew would say, "that hurts."

"Just a few more seconds, Andrew."

Then Scott noticed something: Andrew's thumb had stretched back slightly more.

"Andrew," he said, "look at that. Last week your thumb wouldn't go this far."

It got Andrew's attention.

"You can push it back again."

"Doesn't it hurt?"

"It's okay, Dad."

His fingers began to show slight improvement. Others couldn't tell, but Scott and Andrew saw it.

The Batesons were at an outdoor event downtown and lost sight of Erin in the crowd. Scott snapped at Rebecca: "Where is she?" It took Rebecca by surprise that he would bark at her in public that way, but she didn't say anything about it.

Scott knew he wasn't making an effort with Rebecca, but he felt that was sometimes okay in a marriage—it's one place where you don't have to put on a front. You can give your spouse more of who you are, put more on them than anybody else. That was how he saw it.

Rebecca began to wonder if she could continue to live with Scott this way. It occurred to her that Scott might have some depression, but she was past the point of sympathizing, given how she got the brunt of it. It was easier to continue pushing away.

She felt awkward kissing him good-bye in the morning. Sometimes sitting on the same couch wasn't comfortable. Forget about holding hands. She went to bed clinging to the edge of the mattress. Many nights she fell asleep in the kids' rooms.

Dr. Ginger Manzo walked over from psychiatry to see the Batesons in rehab. She had met the family two months before in intensive care. Back then, her concern had been the mental state of the parents. Now they had asked if she might help with Andrew. He had some new issues lately, Scott said. He had trouble falling asleep, and wanted his parents at night. He had frequent questions about his illness, and his legs. He wanted to know where they were. In a graveyard? No? Then where? It was hard to figure out how much detail to give.

Such questions, Dr. Manzo told Scott, may seem freaky, but they were normal. If Andrew could ask where his legs were without falling apart, that showed good coping skills. Were there other issues?

Yes, tantrums. He would lose his temper if he couldn't have something his way. He had also begun dating things by before and after. There was no more "last summer," or "last winter." It was all pre- or post-operation. He would point to an old drawing: "That's from before I lost my legs." Mention Little League, and you got a similar response. He seemed matter-of-fact about it, but it made the parents sad every time.

Dr. Manzo remembered the first talk she'd had with Andrew. It was just after he'd moved to the fifth floor. "I'm a doctor who helps kids and their families when they've gone through a really hard time," she'd said. "And if you want, you can come talk to me about how you're doing."

Andrew had nodded shyly. The Batesons never pursued it. Now they asked if Andrew could have some sessions. They set up a time.

Rebecca wheeled him into the office, then waited outside. Dr. Manzo had plenty of toys; as soon as Andrew saw them, he wanted to get out of his chair. Manzo felt a bit awkward unbuckling him, which was silly, since she was a physician, but she had no experience moving a bilateral amputee.

She sat on the floor too. She wore slacks and a shirt, and had long brown hair.

While Andrew played, Dr. Manzo chatted with him. How was he feeling?

"Pretty good."

Not grumpy or grouchy?

"No." He told her about his Harley-Davidson stuff.

She probed for signs of post-traumatic stress disorder, such as flashbacks, fatigue, nightmares. She didn't come up with much. In the two weeks since she had talked to Scott, Andrew's sleeping problems had improved. He had less need for Mom and Dad to be there at night. He seemed to be functioning better.

Was Andrew thinking a lot about what had happened?

"No."

Did little things scare or startle him?

"Nope." He began to ask questions of Dr. Manzo. When did she first see him?

In the hospital.

Where? Intensive care?

Yes.

He asked if she had kids. Boys or girls? How old? Did she play with them? It was as if he were testing to see if she was child-qualified.

Dr. Manzo asked what happened when he first got sick.

He remembered being in a park, then going home to bed. He remembered being in the car, his dad driving fast. He remembered his parents arguing about whether they should have gotten an ambulance. That was about it.

Then he said: "If I went in an ambulance, maybe I'd still have my legs."

Dr. Manzo told him that wasn't true. Had they waited for an ambulance, things would have taken longer. Dr. Manzo sensed that that registered with him.

Andrew's play was clearly trauma-related. He would pick up an ambulance and some action figures and start a story about someone being taken to the hospital.

"Why?" Dr. Manzo asked. "What happened?"

"Because they're getting all chopped up."

That idea, multiple amputations, came in over and over.

At a later session with the parents, Scott asked Dr. Manzo why Andrew was playing that way.

"That's what he's thinking about," explained Manzo.

At that, Scott told her how, at home, Andrew would say, "Hey, Dad," and draw a fake knife across his throat or upper arm. It freaked Scott out, but Andrew did it with a humorous look.

Dr. Manzo thought it wasn't a bad sign. It told her Andrew was thinking about his trauma daily, but handling it well.

The parents told Dr. Manzo that Andrew sometimes spoke of an imaginary friend, a tough, cool guy who drove a motorcycle and had a black leather jacket. Dr. Manzo felt that if Andrew was going to have such a friend, that was a good choice—someone strong and cool. Better than a more infantile object of identification.

Dr. Manzo was surprised that Andrew let things out so quickly and blatantly. He never built with blocks or had an army battle. He just began right in with siren sounds and people put into an ambulance. Almost always it was about some accident resulting in limb loss.

"What's happening to these people?" Dr. Manzo asked.

"They got their legs and arms chopped off." Usually it was more extensive than his own injury.

She asked where their legs and arms were.

He'd point to the ceiling. "Up there."

"Where's up there?"

"I don't know."

That seemed to be a question on his mind, wondering what had become of his legs.

Kids often had violence in their play, but Andrew's focus on limb loss was not developmentally normal. Just the same, Dr. Manzo considered it a healthy response to his specific trauma; he could look straight at it. Andrew seemed to understand what these sessions were for.

A few times he worked it out on paper. Dr. Manzo felt that a psychiatrist shouldn't interpret every drawing as having hidden meaning, but with Andrew you couldn't help it. He once drew a bunch of colors next to each other. "It's a rainbow," he said. Then he drew a big black line through the middle, cutting it in half. During one session, he had some drawing paper in his hands and began to rip it. As he did, he said, "Chop, chop, chop." He got obsessive about it and seemed stressed. That was one time Dr. Manzo broke him out of the pattern.

"Okay, okay," she said. "Slow down. What's getting chopped?"

No answer. That was all right. This was part of working things out.

From time to time, Dr. Manzo dropped by rehab at Hasbro to say hello. Once Andrew came out of the pool with a squeeze toy full of water and let her have it. He did it with a look that said, "Can you handle this?" It was a little fresh, but Dr. Manzo didn't mind. Andrew was quite impish.

The parents told her that at home, Andrew was asking how he got sick, and why, and would he get sick again if they went back to that park?

The Batesons could have told him, "Let's not think about that." But they never changed the subject, as some parents might have. Dr. Manzo thought Scott and Rebecca offered honest, age-appropriate answers. She gave them credit for that. Children, she thought, were better off hearing the truth about hard things. Whether it was a parent's death or this, Manzo believed that avoidance prolonged grieving.

Dr. Manzo found herself thinking about other reasons Andrew seemed resilient. For one, his mom and dad had forged a good attachment with him before he got sick. Manzo considered this a predictive factor of how well a child coped with stress. For another, the Batesons' ability to build close friendships gave Andrew a supportive community.

Manzo did not find the parents in sync on everything. When it came to hand-stretching at home, Scott was more persistent. They also were at odds with the rehabilitation people about what limits to set. Rebecca tended to be more lenient.

Andrew told Dr. Manzo that his parents occasionally argued. He said his dad sometimes seemed mad, though not at him or Erin. He felt his dad was mad at his mom, somewhat.

He didn't say this with distress. Somehow, he could tell things were stable between his parents. At least that was his perception.

Manzo did pick up on tension between Scott and Rebecca; you didn't need to be a psychiatrist to see it.

After one session, Andrew settled into the waiting area while Rebecca came inside.

"Andrew seems to be doing okay," Manzo said. "How are you and Scott doing?"

Rebecca said it wasn't a priority right now. Manzo told her that if a marriage doesn't make it, the child often feels responsible. She didn't want that to happen to Andrew.

Rebecca didn't think Andrew was aware of friction; Scott's anger mostly came her way. Frankly, added Rebecca, Scott himself probably didn't think there was a marriage problem.

Perhaps, said Manzo, her office could be a place for the Batesons to talk about things.

Rebecca didn't think she was up to it. She was sure Scott wouldn't be. Nor did she have time. They were doing close to forty hours a week of physical therapy.

After a later session, Dr. Manzo brought both parents into her office. She asked again about their marriage. Had they talked about it with a counselor?

No. They hadn't.

Manzo didn't believe in forcing therapy on people, but she did say she worried about Rebecca and Scott—for Andrew's sake. It would be harder for him to recover if the two of them weren't together.

Scott shifted in his seat. "I just don't want to deal with that," he said. "I don't want to talk about it."

Rebecca shook her head, as if to say, *You see, Doctor?*

Scott's dynamic was familiar to Dr. Manzo. When a child is sick, many parents are unable to deal with anything but that. Andrew's issues were overwhelming enough. For Scott and Rebecca to start talking about "us" felt exhausting to him, and indulgent.

Manzo worried that they could end up separating at some point. It happened often after a trauma involving a son or daughter. It was a dangerous thing in a marriage. A child's illness often led to parents putting each other second and then ignoring the fallout.

After a half dozen sessions, Dr. Manzo noticed that Andrew's action figures recovered with their limbs reattached. To her, that showed resolution and hope. Occasionally he even started playing simple games with stuffed animals that had nothing to do with any accident.

Out of the blue, Andrew asked Dr. Manzo, "If I hadn't lost my legs, would I be coming here to see you?"

"No, Andrew, probably not."

He looked at her and said, "I don't want to come anymore."

"Okay. You don't have to if you don't want to. You can if you do, but it's up to you, Andrew."

Afterward, Manzo mentioned it to Scott. It surprised him. Andrew just came out and said that?

In one way, Dr. Manzo thought it was early for Andrew to stop. They'd had only ten sessions, and she didn't think they were done. But Andrew did. Perhaps he was right. He had sped along at his own pace and gotten it done. He seemed driven to get back to a normal life. Basically, he fired her. She couldn't color it any other way.

Dr. Manzo told the Batesons she thought he would get better faster than they expected.

Just in case, she tentatively scheduled another appointment. She told the parents to come back only if Andrew wanted to. She hoped he would; she liked the idea of keeping up with him. She doubted that Andrew would change his mind, though. And he didn't.

Chapter 14

"The class has been waiting for you . . ."

Rebecca and Scott drove Andrew three blocks to the Kennedy School in Providence. It was just after February vacation, in 1998. It would be his first day back since falling ill the previous July. His class, now first grade, had done most of the year without him. The parents took the wheelchair from the car and helped Andrew into it. As Rebecca pushed him through the schoolyard, she remembered kindergarten the year before. During drop-offs, Andrew wouldn't let go of her hand. She almost had to pry her way free. She had tried everything to make good-byes easier, like breaking a twig and putting half in each of their pockets. Nothing worked. Andrew would keep his eyes right on Mom until the teacher nudged him into the building.

Now they were back. Rebecca steered his wheelchair down the hall to the classroom. They were not sure how the students would react. She knocked on the door.

Months earlier, Rebecca had arranged for Mrs. Pinksaw, Andrew's kindergarten teacher, to home-tutor him. Rebecca didn't want him held back a grade. Two afternoons a week, Andrew and Mrs. Pinksaw sat at the kitchen table, doing math and reading. The sessions started about the time the other kids on the block got home. Andrew could hear them playing outside, and kept turning to look.

Mrs. Pinksaw brought M&M's, but he was still fidgety. He would ask for a drink, for this, for that, to go to the bathroom. Sometimes he put his head on the table. Mrs. Pinksaw didn't blame him; Andrew was quite weak. He could barely hold a pencil.

At one point he kept reaching toward his foot. Mrs. Pinksaw asked what the problem was. He said his ankle itched. Could she scratch it for him? Mrs. Pinksaw didn't know how to react at first. Then she saw that smile; he was messing with her. Mrs. Pinksaw referred to it as the Andrew Look. It got him out of a lot of mischief. It didn't always work, but sometimes it did.

In December Rebecca shared something with Mrs. Pinksaw: She and Scott had been talking with Andrew about Christmas. "I'm going to ask Santa Claus for my legs back," he had said. Mrs. Pinksaw hadn't heard him express such thoughts before. She doubted it was something he dwelt on often. Still, it kind of broke her heart. He had just turned seven.

Rebecca asked Andrew what book he wanted her to read him for bedtime. He chose *Guess How Much I Love You*. He often picked that book—the same one she used to read him when he was in a coma. Rebecca thought it had to be more than coincidence. It wasn't his only mention of things that had happened when he was under. Once Andrew said he remembered Aunt Deb drinking iced tea in the hospital. "I was so thirsty," he said, "I was just looking at her." Rebecca realized he had been unconscious at the time. Lately he had been telling his mother he hated pink soap. Rebecca didn't understand that one; then it came up on a visit to the PICU, and Claire Piette figured it out. The brushes they had used for the early dressing changes, before he woke up, had pink soap in them. Maybe, thought Rebecca, the nurses were right about comas; certain things did register.

Deb Powers was home when Andrew called. Could he talk to Uncle Steve? She handed the phone to her husband. Andrew asked when they were going to see *George of the Jungle*. Months before,

Steve had promised to take him to it. Steve didn't think anything of it since Andrew had been comatose, so it was surprising to hear him bring it up now. Anyway, Steve gave Rebecca a date and said he'd come by to take Andrew.

Steve worried whether he could handle the situation. "You'll just do it," said Deb. Steve had been married long enough to know that was the end of the discussion. When the time came, he carried Andrew to and from the car, and to and from his seat in the theater. It worked out. Andrew didn't seem at all self-conscious.

Much of each day, it was just Rebecca and Andrew.

"Mom," he said, "Mom, Mommy, could you get me my motorcycles?" She was in the middle of picking up from breakfast. She went upstairs to get what he wanted and came down, and he was saying it again.

"Mom. Mom? Mommy?"

"I'm coming."

"Could you get me the Legos?"

"I thought you wanted your motorcycles."

"I changed my mind."

By January, four months after he had come home, Rebecca was thinking Andrew might need a break from Mom. Or maybe it was she who needed the break. She was beginning to feel like a hired hand.

Rebecca asked the school principal, Eileen Koshgarian, if Andrew could rejoin his class a few hours a week. Mrs. Koshgarian said that technically, Andrew would need an IEP, a 504, and a CNA—which, translated, meant an individualized educational plan, a medical plan, and a certified nursing assistant. Such things had to be processed through the state, which would take a while. It would also lock Andrew into a specific schedule, having to report at regular times. Rebecca worried that that could be a problem. Depending on his condition and therapy, Andrew might be in school only a few days each week.

"Rebecca," assured Mrs. Koshgarian, "we'll just work it out." No need, she said, for the alphabet-soup formalities. As far as the school was concerned, Andrew would continue to be home-tutored. If, occasionally, that didn't exactly happen at home, well, no need to bother everyone with such details.

Rebecca and Scott knocked on the door of Andrew's first-grade room. Mrs. Doris McElroy opened it. The children all looked. "Andrew," said Mrs. McElroy, "the class has been waiting for you." Rebecca carried him to his seat and told him Mom and Dad would be nearby. The parents then retreated to the library. They stayed there for perhaps forty-five seconds, then walked back to the class-room. Rebecca stood on tiptoes and peered through the door window. That was how she spent the next hour. The janitor walked by a couple of times and kind of chuckled.

Mrs. McElroy had told her students that Andrew had been very sick, and one of the side effects was that he lost his legs. She didn't make a whole to-do about it. A few of the kids said they knew. Most had gone to kindergarten with him. When Rebecca carried him in, she saw a big banner that said WELCOME BACK ANDREW. Everyone said things like "Andrew's here." None of the kids commented about his legs. It didn't seem to be an issue for them.

Andrew came to class twice a week, an hour or two each visit. Mrs. McElroy often noticed Rebecca at the door. She thought it better not to invite her in, so she pretended not to see.

Pretty soon Rebecca approached the principal and said, "You had better give me something to do." Mrs. Koshgarian was glad to hand her a stack of parent surveys to organize. Mrs. McElroy felt that helped. Andrew was more independent when he didn't see Mom peering in.

On some days, Dad brought him. Scott peered in less. He was concerned but, being a dad, was more low-key about showing it.

...

Andrew began using crutches. A month after that, he was often walking. The stairs, though, were tough. If he felt unsteady on them, he took Mrs. McElroy's hand, which was unusual. She didn't say anything, just quietly went along. Andrew was more public with Mom. When Rebecca came to get him after school, he was happy for her to carry him out. Mrs. McElroy supposed that was the difference between your mom and your teacher.

If Andrew had any anxieties about what people thought, he didn't show it. The only thing Mrs. McElroy noticed was that on stairs, he let other kids pass. He didn't like somebody having to wait for him. Occasionally someone from another class asked, "What happened to you?"

Andrew just said, "I was sick. I had meningitis."

Andrew began therapeutic riding lessons at a country stable called Greenlock. Other kids there had spinal-cord injuries and cerebral palsy. Sometimes that left Rebecca counting her blessings. During one session, Andrew bumped one of his release buttons against the saddle and the leg fell into the dirt. It didn't faze him. He just asked if they could get it. A staffer picked it up and brushed it off. They were very good. Over the weeks, it happened a few more times. Eventually, the Batesons had the prosthetic shop move the button from the side to the back.

Rebecca and Scott grew cautious about certain things. At communion, they took a pass on the wine. Three hundred people drank out of that cup; that was a lot of germs.

It was hard for Rebecca to say yes when Erin asked to sleep at a friend's. What if there were symptoms at night and nobody caught them?

When Rebecca cleaned the house, she began by pouring full-strength Clorox into a spray bottle. In the past she had used Fantastik, but now it had to be bleach. She sprayed it on every tabletop, surface, and doorknob. She used it throughout the bathroom. She took the toothbrushes out of the ceramic wall-holder and cleaned them with hot water. Then she bleached the holder. She stripped the beds and put the pillows in the washing machine. For each load, she added extra bleach. If Rebecca could have made a holster for that spray bottle, she would have. She couldn't scrub the house enough.

Andrew had long wanted an earring and tattoo. Rebecca wasn't sure why, since neither she nor Scott had a wild side. Though maybe that explained it. Andrew had lobbied hardest for the earring, starting at age four. Rebecca told him it was out of the question. While in the PICU, she regretted having said no. She now doubted it would come up again; there was no way Andrew would want to go near a needle if he could help it. But on a mall visit they saw a girl getting her ears pierced inside Claire's, and Andrew asked if he could too.

He would let someone put a needle in him?

Yeah, Mom. Please?

Rebecca had to ask which was the usual side for boys. They told her the left. Were they sure? She didn't want him wearing it on the side that might have meant something. They assured her that the left was fine. Andrew did not even flinch. As far as tattoos, she held the line on that. He had to settle for the ones you got off the label of ravioli cans. Andrew wore those a lot, though not in a normal kid place, like the arm, preferring them on his chest.

In Mrs. McElroy's experience, boys weren't the neatest writers, but Andrew had a particular problem. He gripped a pencil straight up rather than at an angle. He was unable to use his last three fingers, which seemed arthritic.

He also had a problem with cutting; the hand strength wasn't there. Mrs. McElroy had to hold the paper for him. With each month, that got better. As for writing, he was still sloppy but began to use all his fingers.

During recess, Andrew was soon out there trying to run with the best of them. It made Mrs. McElroy nervous. If neither Rebecca nor Scott were there, she kept a close eye. Mrs. McElroy knew that children can fall, but Andrew was a different story. Once or twice he did take a good tumble. She was relieved when he got right back up.

One day the class went to Colt State Park. Mrs. McElroy turned around and there was Andrew, standing on a picnic table. He had that twinkle in his eye, as if to say "Look what I can do." Mrs. McElroy told him to get right down. He did, but was obviously proud of himself. It rattled Mrs. McElroy a bit. What if he had toppled over? Then again, a part of her believed it was a good sign; Andrew was still being Andrew.

Mrs. McElroy was Catholic and strong in her faith. She went to church regularly. In her prayers, she asked God to watch out for Andrew. The way she saw it, who better to talk to about it than the good Lord?

Every so often, Andrew developed a bump or swelling near his knee. It changed everything. Walking became painful, and he wouldn't want to go to school. At one point Andrew got a leg infection. Prosthetics were out of the question. It went on for days, and took the wind right out of Rebecca. It got Andrew down too. They were soaking his knee in the tub when he asked his mother why she let them take his legs. It was his first mention of it in months.

"If we could have," said Rebecca, "Mom and Dad would have had them take our legs instead."

That got his attention.

"How come?"

"Because we'd rather have it happen to us than you. That's the way moms and dads are."

"Oh."

Andrew often brought that back up, usually when in the tub.

"Do you still wish they'd have taken your legs instead of mine?"

"Yes, I do."

Then he switched subjects: "I got to find more kids who don't know much about Pokémon cards."

Why?

"So I can get a good trade."

Scott continued hand-stretching exercises with Andrew. They had started in July of 1997, while he was still in a coma. By the spring of 1998, Andrew had regained almost full hand function. His doctors, including Monica Kleinman, had not expected him to come that far back. She doubted he would have, had it not been for those sessions with his dad.

Scott had worried that Andrew would be affected neurologically by the illness. It turned out not to be the case. Despite his writing issues, Andrew had no problem advancing to the second grade.

That same spring, Scott found a new job and career, as a chemical technician with Dryvit, a company making an exterior finish somewhat like stucco.

Eventually, Rebecca would get a job as a secretary at St. Pius, the neighborhood church whose congregation had prayed so hard for Andrew.

In mid-1998, Rebecca's sisters took her to dinner. It was a year or so since Andrew got home from the hospital. They went to Applebee's.

They asked Rebecca if things were going okay at home.

Things were fine, she said.

"What's really up?" asked Janice.

Rebecca saw no point in denying; these were her sisters. Yes, there were problems. Both she and Scott had pulled away from each other. There were a lot of walls. It had been that way for a while.

"Scott seems angry," Deb said. And short with you.

It surprised Rebecca that her sisters had picked this up. She had thought things looked fine from the outside. She wondered now whether her kids could see it too.

The sisters asked what they could do. Did Rebecca want one of them to talk to Scott? Or the brothers-in-law to do so?

Rebecca didn't think that would work.

Did the two of them need some distance? A separation?

Rebecca nodded. She had thought often about it herself. It might be the best way to help the marriage. She felt there was still a foundation there. Maybe the perspective of living apart—or the shock of it—could get them back to where they used to be. Of course, it might also push them farther apart. But mostly, separating would be a relief.

"Why don't you ask him to leave?"

She doubted he would want to. Scott adored the children. "I don't know how that's going to happen," Rebecca said.

When they left, the sisters told her they were there for her.

"But there's no room at my house," added Janice.

They all had a laugh over that.

If other people had caught on, Rebecca assumed that Andrew and Erin had too—at least on some level. The last thing she wanted was for her kids to worry about how Mom and Dad were. The dinner with her sisters convinced her to finally talk about this with Scott. She told herself she would do it that week. But she couldn't find the right time. There wasn't a right time the next week, either. Months went by, and then more months.

After school got out in June, Mrs. Pinksaw invited the Batesons down to Newport for dinner. Afterwards, they went for a walk on the beach. Mrs. Pinksaw's daughter climbed a lifeguard tower. Then Andrew climbed it.

"Look at him up there," Mrs. Pinksaw's husband said to her. "That's amazing."

"Well," she said, "he's got that spunk." To her, that was Andrew.

. . .

They began to have some warm days. Andrew told his parents he wanted to wear shorts. Scott wasn't all that keen on the idea; he said that people might, well, you know, notice or something.

Andrew said he didn't care. He just wanted to wear shorts. Scott realized it was his own issue, not Andrew's.

Erin had a children's class at the Rhode Island School of Design. Rebecca told Andrew to put his legs on.

He didn't want to.

"Honey, there's going to be lots of people."

So?

She had to admit it bothered her more than him. Andrew didn't focus much on what others thought. Rebecca wished she knew where that came from; she would have bottled it and given it away. She scooped him up and off they went.

Rhonda Mullen from across the street took Andrew and some others to a nearby park. While playing, the catch on one leg released, and off it came. A little girl kept gawking. Andrew finally asked what she was looking at. She didn't answer.

"I have a fake leg," he told her.

She asked how come.

"I got meningitis and I got fake legs."

She didn't seem to know what to say to that. To Rhonda, Andrew's attitude was "So much for her," and he went back to playing.

Another time, the Batesons were at the beach with a group of friends. One of the kids, a little boy, couldn't stop asking Andrew questions. Where did he get the fake legs? How did they work? Did he like them?

The boy's mom asked Rebecca if she should tell him to stop.

No, let it go. Andrew would handle it.

Finally, Andrew pointed at some other child sitting on the beach. "See that boy?" Andrew said. "He's got fake legs too." The other boy didn't, but it was Andrew's way of getting out from under.

Pete Lovegreen, a bartender in Providence, was a friend of the family. A customer heard him talking about Andrew. Then and there, the customer said he wanted to give the family a trip to Walt Disney World. Pete wasn't sure how to take it, but it proved for real.

A limousine picked up the Batesons for the ride to Logan Airport in Boston. There were two connecting rooms waiting for them at the Grand Floridian. It was so unlike the Batesons' usual hotel setup that the kids called it "our apartment."

Andrew walked the parks in shorts. Many folks stared, then looked away if caught. Rebecca realized she used to do the same thing around people who were different. Now it felt insulting, like folks first wanted to gawk at Andrew, then make him disappear. Rebecca encouraged Andrew to smile and say hi. It seemed to make them more comfortable.

While in line, a few politely asked what had happened to Andrew, which was fine with Rebecca. "Well," she said, "he got meningitis." Most were shocked. They never knew that could happen.

At day's end, Andrew was in the pool at the Grand Floridian. Rebecca, who was in a lounger, heard him say, "Hey Dad, my leg fell off." It floated to the surface, looking like a normal leg with its cosmetic covering. As Scott went to retrieve it, people moved away. A few kids got out of the pool. It vaguely reminded Rebecca of a scene from *Jaws*. Scott got Andrew into a chair, reattached the leg, and took him back in. By then, everyone had figured it out. Rebecca thought it was the kind of moment that gave people perspective.

They were there eight days, and everything was paid for. The donor's only request was that the Batesons get him a picture of Andrew with Mickey. They had to pass it along by way of the bartender, so the man could stay anonymous.

. . .

Andrew's parents bought him a battery-powered four-wheel car big enough for a kid to drive. He liked to take it up and down the sidewalk on College Road. The other kids would run next to him. Joe Mullen, the painter from across the street, never got tired of watching that. It was too bad Andrew couldn't ride a regular bike, but the way Mullen saw it, the community came together for this child. Everybody and anybody. Mullen choked up a bit when he thought about it.

Chapter 15

"Did I just see Andrew go down the sidewalk?"

A ndrew kept asking his parents about his bike. He was still too small for the Harley look-alike model, so they hauled up a little yellow one he used to ride. Scott brought it to the sidewalk and held Andrew on its seat. Andrew tried the pedals, but his prosthetic feet slipped off them. All he could do was sit, and only for a few minutes. He gave up and said, "I'll never be able to do this." Rebecca remembered how, when he was only four, he asked them to remove the training wheels. As soon as they did, off he went. That was typical. One thing Scott and Rebecca never had to do was coax Andrew to stay with a sport. A book, maybe.

Rebecca felt discouraged as they put the bike away. She did not feel Andrew would be able to ride again.

But he kept wanting to try. They walked him on the bike three or four times a week. Rebecca considered it a bad idea. She felt that they were setting him up for failure. She thought about getting him a tricycle like the one in therapy. It would be the right bike, but she worried that it would give him the wrong message. So Andrew kept at the two-wheeler.

He learned to sit on it unbraced, his legs dangling to either side for balance. Then he said he wanted to coast. His parents resisted, but Andrew kept asking. Finally, Rebecca and Scott stood a few feet apart, one giving Andrew a light push. He rolled free for a second or so. The other caught the bike and sent him back. It became a regular thing. Scott and Rebecca were soon standing ten feet apart, Andrew coasting between them.

He still could not pedal. Rebecca thought: *How could you, with feet you can't feel?* She considered strapping them on, but decided against it. Talk about a setup for a fall.

College Road had a downhill grade. Andrew wanted to coast on his own with no parent to catch him. Scott put a helmet and elbow pads on Andrew, and pointed him. "Let go," Andrew said. Scott did. Nearby, Rebecca was biting her lip. Andrew wavered, but soon he was doing it. Then he swerved into a driveway, fell hard, and started to cry. Scott reached him pretty quickly. He had banged his knee.

"I can't ride my bike, Dad," Andrew said. "I can't ride it anymore."

"It's going to take time," Scott said. Andrew told him just to put it away.

A week later, he was outside preparing to coast again. Scott let go, then hustled to keep pace alongside. He couldn't let Andrew fall; that last one had really been a setback. Andrew was a bit shaky, but he held it, coming to a stop on his own. Later, Scott stood near Rhonda Mullen, talking about how afraid he was that Andrew would crash. "He's going to," said Rhonda. "Kids fall even if they don't have fake legs." Scott wished he could look at it that way.

Andrew found he could practice on his own if he used the picket fence in front of the house for support. Rebecca watched as he pushed off, coasted a few yards, then grabbed the wood. At one point he got his elbow stuck between pickets, which gave Rebecca a start. He was out there over an hour. Rebecca wished he wasn't so obsessive. It would make her job a lot easier.

Now that he'd figured out the fence technique, Andrew began

practicing almost every day. Soon he was gliding a few yards past the fence, then putting his legs down for a safe stop. Often, Rebecca was the one running behind him. She was more prone than Scott to grab the back of his bike. Andrew didn't like that. He tried the pedals, but his feet slid off. He kept trying, though. Andrew seemed determined to ride a two-wheeler. For months, he just kept at it.

Scott pulled home from work, and before he even got out of his car Andrew was at his window.

"Dad, I want to try my bike."

Neighborhood kids were out riding, too. That was often what got Andrew going; he wanted to do whatever he was looking at. Scott got him suited up. Rebecca came outside and watched as Scott pushed Andrew downhill. He briefly coasted, then tried to pedal. This time his feet did not slip. He continued down the sidewalk, past one house, two, three. Andrew was riding his bike.

Then he bumped the button on one of his prosthetics, and his leg fell to the concrete. Scott yelled for Joseph Mullen, a neighborhood boy who was nearby, to catch Andrew. Joseph chased him and grabbed the bike. Scott went running down the street toward Andrew too.

A moment before Andrew's leg came off, a college-aged jogger had come around the corner. He saw the whole thing and appeared panicked. He asked if they wanted him to call 911. Scott didn't have time to chat about it. He just grabbed Andrew's detached leg and kept running. The young man looked as though he had seen a ghost. His face was white, and he appeared to be shaking. Rebecca thought he was definitely in the wrong place at the wrong time. He kept glancing back at the people around Andrew as he continued on his way. Scott still had Andrew's leg in his hand.

Afterward, Scott would joke about the college student who perhaps still thought he saw a child get his leg sliced off by a bike. At the same time, Scott felt bad for the young man. It was not the kind of sight you would easily get over. The next day, Scott and Rebecca decided to get Andrew a bike with handbrakes.

. . .

Andrew had played T-ball the year before, and wanted to step up to Little League. Rebecca considered it a bad idea. It would only show Andrew how different he was. Running, Scott admitted, was quite a challenge for a bilateral.

"Hon," said Rebecca, "maybe this year we might try something else."

But all his friends played, said Andrew.

She told him Little League was different than T-ball.

So?

Later, Scott mentioned it to a friend, who wondered whether Andrew was pushing himself too hard. Perhaps the boy was putting pressure on himself. Scott didn't see it that way. In the end, Andrew was a pretty simple kid. It wasn't that he felt he should; he just wanted to. Scott signed him up.

The one concern Andrew mentioned was striking out. Scott had expected the opposite worry: getting a hit and having to run. Or having to chase a ball in the field. But those things didn't come up.

Rebecca was unable to make Andrew's first game. When he and Scott got home, she did her best to sound supportive.

"How many points did you get?" she asked.

"They're not points, Mom," said Andrew, "they're runs."

Scott had expected the running issue to demoralize his son, but the only time it came up was when Andrew mentioned a teammate who also had a disability. Andrew told his father, "I might have to run for him because he has trouble." Scott wondered if Andrew was kidding. Later, Andrew said it again.

"We'll let the coach worry about that," said Scott.

Andrew hung in there, but he didn't seem to love baseball. Rebecca felt that the problem wasn't running; it was downtime. Between the dugout and the field, there was too much waiting. Andrew liked constant action. That, thought Rebecca, had been his pace from day one. He never was one to sit still. Even in the bathtub he practiced his throw with a washcloth.

Andrew's next thing was joining a basketball league. It took his father by surprise. Had Scott been the one with two prosthetic legs, he would not have attempted such a game. He allowed his son to try, but wasn't sure how it would work. The basketball coach found a way. He set Andrew up under the other basket. The kids passed him the ball, and he shot. He missed his share, but he did put a few in. Rebecca felt it took some gumption to put himself in the hot seat that way.

It reminded her of Andrew's old personality. It had really stood out that time in Story Land in New Hampshire, where they'd gone before Andrew got sick. While Erin bit her fingernails, Andrew was up for everything. The flume, the roller coaster, you name it. He kept pulling at his parents, saying, "Let's go." He was even that way about food. Rebecca couldn't get her daughter to try a clam if her life depended on it. Andrew put one right in his mouth. He immediately spit it back out at her, but he tried it. That was Andrew; he had to try everything.

The Batesons got a phone message from A-Wish-Come-True. Someone had submitted Andrew's name and Rebecca was touched, but it kind of unsettled her. A-Wish-Come-True, she felt, was for terminally ill children. She didn't call back, even though they left several messages. In late September they finally reached her.

Rebecca thanked them but said Andrew didn't qualify.

Why was that?

Because he was fine now.

Children, she was told, don't have to be terminal. They just need to have a life-threatening illness.

Soon after, a planner for the group came by the Batesons' home. If you could have anything you'd like, she said to Andrew, what would it be?

He didn't have to think about his answer.

"A pool," he said.

Rebecca hadn't seen that one coming. She had never considered it; their backyard was too small. But a pool company donated an aboveground model that just barely fit.

Andrew was not able to wear his latest pair of legs into the pool. The coverings were too spongy, and the insides prone to rust. Ideally, he needed a new pair of specially made water-legs, which were hollow. He had outgrown the makeshift ones he had gotten for the therapy pool. But now the insurance company said no. They considered it a luxury. Rebecca felt that might be the case if you were a unilateral, but it was different for a bilateral. Without them, Andrew could neither jump off the side nor touch bottom.

Rebecca decided to have them made while appealing the decision. When the legs were done, the caseworker called Rebecca back. She had tried hard, but the company had rejected the claim. The Batesons had to pay the full $9,000 cost. It was their first insurance rejection. Had it not been for the fund-raisers, Rebecca wasn't sure what they would have done.

The people at A-Wish-Come-True learned about Andrew's Harley obsession. They invited the Batesons to an Elks Lodge for a special event. The Ocean State Harley Owners Group, known as HOGS, was holding a poker ride. The way it worked, bikers paid to join and stopped on the way at five locations to get a playing card. Whoever ended up with the best hand won a prize. The Elks Lodge was the final stop. The proceeds went to A-Wish-Come-True.

Once the riders had arrived, the Batesons walked to the parking lot to look at all the Harleys. Andrew fixated on one in particular. The bike's derby cover was a cast-aluminum skull. So were its cleaner cover, point cover, and rocker cover. The event organizers asked the owner if he might give Andrew a short ride. His name was Bernie Lemire, but his friends called him by his nickname, Skull. He got the name for shaving his head before it was fashionable. He also had a big beard and wore a jean vest with a skull on the back.

Lemire posed with Andrew for a picture, then gave him a ride around the lot. His Harley had aftermarket pipes on it, so it was louder than a stock bike. Andrew didn't seem to have much fear about riding on a noisy motorcycle with a bald and bearded man named Skull. Bernie Lemire was impressed with that.

Lemire did many poker rides each year. He always ended up with weak hands. If he was lucky, he got a pair.

The Batesons invited the Harley people to visit their home. About twenty of them came loudly down College Road, many with wives or girlfriends aboard. Bernie Lemire was among them. They gave Andrew some leather gear and made him an official HOG. Rebecca served soda and snacks. Andrew asked his father to bring up his own Harley bicycle. It looked big for the boy, and Skull Lemire guessed it was for show. But when it came time to leave, Andrew got on it and led the whole contingent—twenty Harleys—down the street. It was nearly dark. Skull hadn't expected Andrew to get around as well as he did. He felt that this was one gutsy kid.

To Rebecca, it was some sight, a little peanut leading all these scary-looking motorcyclists. It was a great afternoon.

Andrew started asking about his Rollerblades. Rebecca's policy was never to discourage him, but with extreme requests it was important to be honest. "Hon," said Rebecca, "I don't know if you're going to be able to do that again." Andrew wanted to try. His first in-line skates, at age four, had been the PlaySkool ones with locking wheels that strapped to shoes. They were a waste of money since Andrew found them too slow. Instead, he talked Erin out of her blades. They were huge, coming up to his knees, but he was soon skating down the sidewalk in them. That had been two years before.

As she went to the basement to get his blades, Rebecca reminded him he did not have his strength back, and—

"Hurry up, Mom."

Putting Rollerblades on artificial legs was a reality check for

Rebecca. It was hard to do, since the prosthetic ankles would not bend. When she was done, she briefly worried she had buckled them too tight, then caught herself. Andrew was unable to stand on his own. Rebecca supported him under his arms from behind, steering him outdoors. They worked their way down the sidewalk, both struggling. Andrew seemed to have no balance or coordination. Were Rebecca to let go, he would have collapsed. Pretty soon he got frustrated. He told his mother just to take his skates off. He wasn't crying openly, but she could hear it in his voice. She sat him down and began to unbuckle the skates. He walked back up the sidewalk in his socks. When they got in the house, Andrew said he didn't think he could ever do this. Rebecca did not want to lead him on. "You might not, honey," she said.

After a few days Andrew wanted to try again. He asked if he had to wear all his gear.

"Yes, Andrew."

Could he at least not wear elbow pads?

"Andrew."

It was an ordeal getting everything on. Again they made their way to the sidewalk.

"Come on, Mommy, let go."

She resisted, but he kept asking, so she did. Andrew fell. He came down hard, began to cry, and wanted everything off. It had taken thirty minutes to get him geared up, but after seconds he was done. When they got back inside, Andrew said that this time he really meant it. He never wanted to go skating again. Rebecca felt it was just as well.

The next week, she was wrestling the skates back onto his feet. Scott often went through the same ritual with him.

Soon Andrew was trying it every few days. He would see other kids skating, and that was how his mind worked. He was not making much progress, though. Then he got the idea of starting on the grass, where he was able to stand on his own. At least that let Rebecca off the hook. Supporting him on blades wasn't easy on the back. Andrew walked on the lawn for a bit, then made it to the sidewalk, gripping the picket fence for support.

Rebecca watched as he rolled, picket by picket. A few times, he half fell but pulled himself up. It seemed like a lot of work. It was 10 A.M. and getting hotter.

Ready to quit, Andrew?

No. He wanted to keep doing this.

"I don't think it's going to work, honey."

It got to be a daily thing. Andrew woke up, had a banana and orange juice, and then wanted his blades on. Rebecca would watch from the house as he walked across the lawn to the picket fence and started in. It was July 3, 1998, and especially hot. Rebecca had not looked forward to that day, the first anniversary of his getting sick. There were a lot of this-time-last-years.

Andrew began to experiment with letting go of the pickets. He fell just about every time. Rebecca went about her business. When she next looked out, she was surprised to see Andrew rolling a few feet, bent at the waist for balance. Then he grabbed the pickets to stop. Once he reached bottom, Andrew pulled himself a step at a time uphill and started again. He never went beyond the fence, which was about twenty feet long.

It dawned on Rebecca that he had been at it over an hour. She asked if he wanted to stop.

No. He was fine.

He continued for yet another hour. By now he had worked up to a few yards before grabbing on. Other kids came by to hang out but drifted away. Andrew stayed at it. Rebecca looked outside every so often. He was either resting on the grass or doing that bent-over glide. A few times he fell on his rear end. It didn't seem to stop him. Truth be told, she was happy that he was keeping himself busy. It gave her a chance to get a few things done around the house.

. . .

"Mom!"

Andrew was calling her. "Mom, watch."

Rebecca sat on the front steps. Andrew let go and began to glide downhill. He skated for two yards, then three. It looked like he was going to coast the whole fence. She waited for him to grab the end. Instead he went past it, continuing down the sidewalk. He went beyond the neighbor's house and turned up the next driveway, rolling to a stop. He was quite unsteady but remained upright. He was sweating, with a proud look on his face.

A few seconds before, Scott had driven onto College Road. It was the end of his workday; that was how long Andrew had been at this. Scott looked out the car window and noticed a child skating.

"Did I just see Andrew go down the sidewalk?" he said as he pulled up to the house.

"You sure did," said Rebecca.

"That's amazing," said Scott. "He's skating."

It was more like gliding, but as far as Rebecca was concerned, if he got no better this was still a big leap. "You did it, Andrew," she said.

That afternoon, Father Ken Letoile stopped by. Rebecca told him what Andrew had done. The following Sunday he commented about it in his homily. Every so often he was prone to do that, give the church an Andrew update.

The next day, July 4, Dr. Monica Kleinman found herself thinking about Andrew. Given all her patients, it was unusual that she would be struck by the anniversary of one of them. She called the family to say hello. Scott told her that Andrew had been biking and playing Little League, even in-line skating. It made her think back to his time in the hospital. She had doubted then that he would ever again be able to throw a ball. She could still picture how dark his fingers had been. Dr. Kleinman considered Andrew a noteworthy case of survival. The strength of the infection in him had been impressive.

It helped that he had received meticulous care, but she thought it also said something about Andrew's biological strength.

Both Bateson kids were invited to a birthday party at United Skates, an indoor roller rink. A few days before, Erin had gotten a bone bruise on her hand, and she arrived with it wrapped. The attendants said she couldn't skate; children with injuries weren't allowed. Erin had to sit and watch. By now Andrew was really skating, pushing off each foot for speed. Erin kept saying it wasn't fair. By rink rules, Andrew shouldn't be allowed to skate either. Talk about an injury—he didn't even have legs. It was hard for Rebecca to explain the difference. Andrew seemed pleased by it all.

Deb Powers gave her sister and brother-in-law a lot of credit. Andrew, she believed, could have been an invalid, but they let him try whatever he wanted to. Rebecca didn't think the compliment was deserved in her case. She'd tried to talk Andrew out of plenty of things, but found she didn't have all that big a say.

Andrew spent much of the summer on wheels of various kinds. He often in-line skated in the house, which Rebecca did not love. Outdoors, he played games of driveway hockey with the other kids. He had a wide stance and an awkward turn, but all Rebecca could say was that it was better than she could do. The driveway hockey occasionally left Andrew frustrated to the point of crying, though not because of his skating ability. It was when the other side kept scoring. Andrew had long had an issue about losing. He still did.

Chapter 16

"That kid has more guts than anyone I've ever seen . . ."

Andrew's second-grade teacher was Mrs. Meg Ford. She was unsure how Andrew would do, it being his first full-time school schedule. Given his prosthetics, she expected him to be shy. The main problem, though, was that he got chatty from time to time. Mrs. Ford called him on it, as she would anyone else. She felt for Andrew, but that didn't mean she was going to let him get away with anything.

Although Mrs. Ford made up her mind to treat him the same as others, his condition did come up. Once Andrew accidentally stepped on her toe. She hadn't realized prosthetics were so heavy. When the class gathered on the rug, only a few kids got to sit in chairs. That was considered a privilege. Mrs. Ford always picked Andrew, as he was unable to sit Indian style. That was about the only way she accommodated him.

The other students barely brought up Andrew's situation, even when he wore shorts. They seemed to see him as Andrew, not as a child without legs. Mrs. Ford didn't know if he would always be that insulated, but he was at the Kennedy School.

The district assigned Andrew a certified nursing assistant. He called her Miss April. At first he held back, which she understood.

It took time for a child to accept a full-time, one-on-one aide. Miss April told herself to be patient. Things would come at their own pace.

A few weeks into the year, the two were sitting together outside the school nurse's office. From time to time, Andrew got headaches. He pushed the release button on one of his prosthetic legs and handed it to Miss April. She held it a moment, and, smiling, offered it back to him.

"Why are you giving this to me?" she asked.

"That doesn't freak you out?" he said.

Miss April was twenty-five years old. As a CNA, she had been around the block. No, it didn't.

"I just took off my leg," said Andrew.

"And . . . is there a point?"

"Did you know I didn't have legs?"

"Yes."

"Oh."

Miss April felt she had been given a test and passed. Afterward, Andrew was more open with her.

Andrew's favorite subject was recess, held in the paved schoolyard. It took time for Miss April to get comfortable with how active he was. He even played tag. The boys usually chased the girls.

At first, Miss April would tell him to slow down. She was afraid he might slip. But Andrew would just say, "Miss April, I'm okay."

Miss April believed that Andrew got his strength from his family's faith. She knew a little about that because of her own sister, who, as a bystander, was struck by a bullet at a party when a shooting broke out. Her sister was left paralyzed from the neck down. They said she wouldn't live past three months, and if she did, she would be on a ventilator. Now she breathed on her own and ate solid food. She could move her shoulders and had regained feeling in one elbow. Miss April believed that God helped heal her. The family had put faith in Him and trusted in His words, because the Bible said that by His stripes we will be healed. Miss April believed

God gave her sister life for some special reason. She believed the same thing about Andrew.

One day at recess, Miss April noticed that a particular kid kept targeting Andrew during tag. Afterward, Andrew sat with her.

"I wish I had my legs so I could run faster," he said. "I'm tired of being It all the time."

Miss April said, "One day you *will* be the fastest, if you keep working at it."

That seemed to make him feel better.

An adult usually stayed near the schoolyard gate at recess to keep balls from the street. That was often Miss April's post. She was standing there when Andrew walked up. She looked at his face and could just tell.

"Is something wrong, Andrew?"

"No."

"Andrew, something's bothering you."

"They won't let me play handball because they said I was too slow." They had teams, he explained, and didn't pick him.

"Do you want me to speak to them?"

"No."

"What do you want to do?"

"Sit down next to you."

She didn't press him. Andrew liked to keep things in. That was how certain children were, thought Miss April. Some things you can't know.

She mentioned it to Mrs. Ford, who later had a class conversation about excluding kids. She kept it general. Mrs. Ford asked everyone to think about how they would feel if left out of something, like a game. The problem pretty much ended after that.

A part of Andrew reminded Mrs. Ford of her husband, Wayne. They had been married for nineteen years. During sixteen of them, he had had cancer. It started in his thymus gland and traveled to his lungs. At first they said he would have only six months.

It was quite a shock. Wayne was still in college then, and Meg asked if he wanted to stop school, but he didn't. Meg felt that was courage—living as normally as possible. The six-month point passed, and Wayne remained healthy enough. The doctors figured radiation had done an exceptional job, but Meg Ford felt God had a hand in it, too. She and Wayne had made Christ the center of their marriage. They trusted that God knew what He was doing, even when they didn't like what was happening one bit. Through Him, they learned to live a day at a time. They took that lesson from Matthew 6:34.

Over the years, the cancer spread here and there. More than a few times, Wayne had to have an operation right away. It was discouraging. Once, when things were very bleak, the two wrote Bible verses on poster board and hung them around the living room. It helped to be literally surrounded by Scripture. Then they prayed each verse back to God. It gave them a lot of comfort.

As Wayne kept surviving, both he and Meg began to think that God was up to something, so they never let a cloud stay over their heads. Wayne earned a master's degree and became a visiting nurse. When they found they couldn't have a baby together, they decided to adopt. When told they couldn't have an infant because of Wayne's illness, they went through the foster system and adopted two school-age children. That proved one of the richest blessings. Their daughter Dawn's junior year was a hard time for Wayne's health, but he made it to all her games. He had his little oxygen tank, and off he went. He was bound and determined to not let this get in the way. If he had, Meg felt they probably wouldn't have had as happy a life. They wouldn't have adopted children and now have grandchildren. But they just took each day, and it turned into nineteen years. Wayne died in 1991 at age forty-three. Meg got through it by staying in Scripture. She didn't understand all the whys, but she trusted in God.

It wasn't as if Mrs. Ford looked at Andrew and always thought of her husband. It was more subconscious than that. But to her the comparison was clear enough: Like Wayne, Andrew just went on normally. He focused on what he had. In that sense, Mrs. Ford identified with his situation.

Several times, Rebecca had to take Erin to the hospital for her asthma. Once she was held overnight. Rebecca stayed, and after a few hours, felt she'd lose it if they didn't get out soon. Then she caught herself. Hadn't she made it through nine weeks? The doctors considered taking Erin to the intensive care unit, but the attack subsided—a big relief to Rebecca. She preferred not to go back inside those walls if she could help it.

Rebecca and Andrew were preparing to leave the hospital's prosthetic department after an adjustment. He asked her why everyone called him a bilateral.

"Because you lost both your legs," said Rebecca. "If you only lost one of your legs, you'd be a unilateral."

"What if I lost three legs?"

Then, said Rebecca, you would be a trilateral.

"Four legs?"

A quadrilateral.

By the time they got to eleven, Rebecca had run out of answers.

They were told they had a ten-dollar co-pay. "Unless you're post-operative," the woman added. Andrew answered that he was not post-operative, he was bilateral. Rebecca was impressed that he could joke about it. She was unable to.

Andrew liked visiting the PICU after his rehab sessions. He had no hesitancy about walking through the double doors to say hello to everyone. They made a fuss over him, and, for his part, Andrew was like a little politician, shaking everyone's hand. It made Karen Zelano, one of the nurses, think how differently her own children acted when brought here. They would stare at the kids in their beds and pull on her hand, wanting to leave. Not Andrew: He strode around both pods to see who was there. In late October he came by dressed as a vampire. To Claire Piette, he was just another little boy getting ready for Halloween. It was a good moment. *You work and work,* she thought, *and then you see them healthy.*

Usually, Rebecca waited outside. She was happy to see the staff, but not the place. Neither did she wait in the parents' lounge. It didn't hold a lot of good memories for her.

A friend at work got to chatting with Scott about youth hockey. The next day the friend brought in a flyer. Being a typical dad, Scott showed it to Andrew. Would he like to learn hockey?

Scott knew Andrew would say yes. That's the way he was. He had been out of the hospital a little over a year.

Rebecca considered hockey a bad idea. She didn't want to burst Andrew's bubble, but she feared he would get hurt. He had only ice-skated once or twice in his life. Andrew told her she worried too much.

In the Edgewood Youth Hockey League, Andrew started at the instructional level. The higher-level house league was for those ready to play games. Andrew asked his father not to tell anyone about his legs; he didn't want to be treated differently. To keep the secret, Scott suited up Andrew at home and walked him into the rink on skate guards. Andrew stepped onto the ice, quickly fell down, and was unable to get up. Scott, who had brought his own skates, helped him. Andrew scuffled around a bit, then fell again. Scott had to keep lifting him. Perhaps, he thought, Rebecca was right about this one. Apparently, ice-skating was a whole different thing from in-line skating. Scott expected Andrew to say he wanted to quit, or at least rest. All he said was, "Dad, help me up."

There were several practices a week. Andrew continued to have problems when he fell. Scott knew he couldn't pick up Andrew forever. The next time he went down, Scott told him to try on his own. Andrew knelt and planted one skate, but it slipped to the side. It kept doing that. Scott helped him halfway up, let go, and bang, both legs splayed out from under.

Rebecca was in the seats watching. Andrew really seemed to be struggling. She thought ice hockey was not a good idea at all.

House league tryouts were coming up, and Andrew said he wanted to make the cut. Instructional was okay, but his main thing in sports was competing.

"You know, Andrew," Scott said, "if you go into the house league and fall down, Dad can't be there." Andrew said he would be fine.

The next practice, Scott was on the other side of the rink, talking to a coach, when Andrew fell. Rebecca was in the seats watching. *Come on, Andrew,* she thought, *you can do it.* Andrew just lay there. He glanced around for his father. Scott wasn't paying attention. Rebecca saw Scott facing the other way and grew annoyed. Why wasn't he looking out for their son? Andrew got to a half kneel, but his skate slid out. He did this four or five times, then another four or five. After a long struggle, it worked. Rebecca started breathing again. She had not realized Scott had looked away on purpose. That was hard for Scott to do, but he felt he had to.

House league tryouts were at the Providence College rink. They put the kids through their paces. Afterward, a coach skated up to Andrew. "You're on the team, buddy," he said. At the time, he was not aware of Andrew's situation.

Andrew was assigned to Coach Ron Martinelli. He was in his late forties and ran an auto-collision estimate business. He did not consider Andrew the best player on the team, but he wasn't the worst, either. He did seem to have problems getting up after a fall.

After a few weeks of team practice, Andrew developed a swollen knee. They put him on antibiotics, but it was a whole month before he could skate again. Scott thought he should let Martinelli know that Andrew hadn't just disappeared. He went to the next session and waited outside the locker room until Martinelli said good-bye to the last kid. The two greeted each other, and Martinelli asked where Andrew had been.

"I came down to talk to you about that," Scott said. Andrew, he explained, had a bruise on his knee. It was really hurting him. He was having a hard time even walking around.

"Really? How'd it happen?"

Scott didn't know how to put it. "Ron, I didn't talk to you about this before. I just didn't see any reason to mention it, but maybe I should have." Andrew, he said, had contracted meningitis, lost both legs below the knee, and was skating with artificial limbs. Martinelli could have fallen on the floor. He kept saying, "You gotta be kidding me."

Having played the game—he still did in adult leagues—Martinelli knew how hard it was. He couldn't imagine being able to skate if you didn't know where each edge of the blade was. He remembered a TV news story about a young man with a prosthetic lower leg who played basketball for Notre Dame. Had Martinelli seen such a story on Andrew playing hockey, he would have thought, *No way; it's a setup.* He considered hockey the hardest of all team sports. Putting a kid with no legs on skates? He would not have accepted such a thing as possible.

He told Scott, "That kid has more guts than anyone I've ever seen on the ice."

Later, from the sound of it, Rebecca wished Scott had had a camera to capture that coach's expression.

Scott asked Martinelli not to spread it around, since Andrew wanted to blend in. To make sure of that, Martinelli didn't tell his two assistant coaches. He did not tell his wife, either. For the next days, on and off, Martinelli found himself shaking his head about it.

Andrew continued to have trouble getting up after a fall. Martinelli wouldn't help. That was how he treated any other kid; he forced them to figure it out themselves. A couple of times, while Andrew struggled, Martinelli could hear some of the mothers in the stands.

"That kid hurt himself," one said. "Why won't they do something?" Martinelli just went about his business.

Andrew never asked for help, at least not from the coach. It kind of inspired Martinelli. Andrew was one determined little guy. Every time he fell Rebecca held her breath. She did that a lot while at the rink.

Martinelli's one concession was to let Scott on the ice at practices and the bench during games, but only in case of an accident. Martinelli pictured someone running into Andrew and a leg flying off. Were that to happen, they would have needed a fifty-five-gallon drum of smelling salts for the fans. All the mothers, he thought, would be passing out.

Dana Weaver, one of the assistant coaches, asked Martinelli why it was taking Andrew so long to stand back up. Shouldn't he have learned by now? Martinelli sat there biting his tongue. He wasn't saying anything.

Scott was watching drills when another assistant coach skated up to Andrew. The coach seemed concerned about Andrew's equipment. He reached down to adjust his shin guards. Andrew wasn't wearing any. Scott watched as the coach felt through Andrew's sock for the shin pad. He looked confused, then gave up and told Andrew to get back into the drill.

The games were on Saturday mornings. Andrew told his father he wanted to wear his legs to bed Friday night.

Why, Andrew?

That way, he could get suited up for hockey the moment he woke.

Oh. Good idea.

Andrew nodded. He didn't want to waste any time.

Rebecca found it difficult to watch Andrew skate. Some of the kids out there were big and had been at this for years. Occasionally, she got headaches during his two-minute shifts. She couldn't wait for the buzzer. Erin didn't like sitting in the stands by her mother. It was embarrassing the way Rebecca screamed whenever Andrew fell.

Once, another player got in front of Andrew and tripped him up. Both went down together in a heap. Andrew got so aggravated he started poking the other kid with his stick. Every time the kid tried to stand up, Andrew knocked him down. Rebecca felt it was no way for her son to behave. She looked around for Scott and saw him nearby in that dugout thing. She yelled for him to make Andrew stop. She said Andrew should go in the penalty box for it. Scott ignored her, just let it go. Eventually, both kids stood and skated off. Rebecca supposed it was some kind of dad deal: they liked their sons to be aggressive. Whenever Andrew mentioned a kid giving him a hard time, say, at a playground, she counseled him to ignore it. Turn around and walk away. "No you don't," Scott would say. "Push him back. Don't let him do that to you."

Usually, Andrew gave 150 percent on the ice, never complained, but once Martinelli noticed him sitting by himself at the end of the bench. He asked what the problem was. Andrew didn't say anything. Then Martinelli saw some tears. Scott walked over and explained that Andrew was down on himself. He felt he wasn't contributing. For the first time, Martinelli got in Andrew's face a bit.

"You wearing a red shirt?" he asked loudly.

Andrew nodded.

"You a member of this team?"

Another nod.

"Then get your tail out with the rest of them where you belong." Andrew did, and his mood seemed to pass.

Martinelli had expected Andrew's dad to be overprotective, but Scott never asked that they go easy on the kid. Martinelli played Andrew at forward, defense—basically everywhere. During the tougher drills Scott just bit his lip. Same during games when Andrew went into the corners, where there were often collisions. Martinelli gave Scott credit for that. Were he the dad it would have put a hole in him, but Scott sucked it up. Martinelli believed that was one reason Andrew didn't feel inferior. Even though he got dealt a bad hand, his family let him try what he wanted.

Scott himself sometimes wondered how Andrew managed to skate. He was on two stilts and couldn't feel his feet. How could anyone play hockey like that? Had it been him, no way he would be out there trying such things. Scott wasn't sure where Andrew got this from.

Scott did notice one odd thing about Andrew's hockey playing: During games, he sometimes streaked off on his own, away from the action, sprinting down the ice. Scott guessed it was about speed. That was Andrew's thing, always had been. On the ice, despite his prosthetics, he could really move,. He liked that feeling.

It reminded Scott of the first time Andrew got on ice skates. He had been five. They had gone skiing at Waterville Valley, which had a rink. Scott took both kids on the ice. Erin, who knew how to skate, was tentative. Andrew, who had never skated and had to lean on a support chair, took off. He got annoyed when Scott skated with him. Dad, he kept saying, quit following me. He didn't want a traffic cop. Across the ice, Erin clung to her mother. Andrew, thought Scott, was just a different kind of kid.

Deb's son, Scott, was at the United States Coast Guard Academy. When he heard his cousin Andrew was playing hockey, he drove home to catch a couple games. Up until then, he and his sister, Beth, had been the only cousins of thirteen who played the game. They had long hoped another would take it up. Kind of funny, Scott Powers thought, that the one who finally did had no legs.

Andrew's prosthetics were designed to last a year, but Andrew needed new ones in four months. He banged them up and occasionally cracked them. They were constantly in the shop. After a while, they were held together by duct tape. The technicians had seldom seen prosthetic legs in such condition. They kept saying to the family, "Boy, he really uses these."

Rebecca was in the house when she saw Katy Wells's mother walking Andrew back across the street. He was limping more than usual.

"We had a little accident," said Mrs. Wells.

"What happened?"

"I broke your son."

Mrs. Wells explained that he had been on her swing set and had leaped off at the top of the arc. Andrew told Mrs. Wells he heard something crack. Rebecca checked the leg. She noticed his ankle bending a weird way. He had snapped the rod where the foot attached. Rebecca thought it ironic that she still had to worry about broken ankles with Andrew.

Rebecca went to get his old legs, which they kept as backups, but couldn't find them. Andrew treated them like shoes; he left them wherever he took them off. Living room? No. Under the bed? No. In the hockey bag? Yes. Andrew put the old ones on, found a smaller pair of sneakers that fit, and went outside to play again.

The family went skating in downtown Providence at the city's open-air ice rink. An attendant told Andrew to slow down. He did so for a few minutes, then got going again and, while moving at a good clip, took a hard spill. He was having more trouble than usual standing, so Scott came over. Had Andrew hurt himself? No, he was fine. Scott checked out his legs, and sure enough, there was a crack. At that point, an attendant skated up and asked if the boy was all right.

"I think he's okay," said Scott. "He just broke his leg." That was all Scott said. The attendant asked if he should call a rescue.

No, said Scott, but was there any tape around? It then occurred to him what the attendant must be thinking, and he explained Andrew's situation.

Scott carried Andrew to a bench. The legs were only a month old and had cost over $10,000, and Andrew had broken one. As it turned out, the rink had no tape, but a friend came by with a roll he used for hockey.

"Andrew," said Scott, "to fix it I have to take it off." Scott doubted Andrew would want to in public, but he told his dad to go ahead. Scott squeezed the crack together hard and began to wrap it. Andrew kept telling him to hurry up, as if Scott were tying his shoe. Finally, Andrew went back out. Attendants were soon warning him to slow down again.

Andrew's hockey team made it to the championship game. Beforehand, Scott told Martinelli it was okay to finally let the secret out. Martinelli was about to go along, but then he had another idea. "You know something," he said. "Let's not do that." The league banquet was coming up. Martinelli had already thought of doing something extra for Andrew. That might be a better time, he said. It was fine with Scott.

Martinelli did, however, clue in his assistant coaches, Dana Weaver and George Butts. He did so with one minute left in the game. Andrew was on the ice. "I got to tell you something," Martinelli said to the two. "I got to tell you why it takes Andrew so long sometimes when he falls." He did not want them repeating this to anyone, but Andrew had had meningitis, and both of his legs were amputated below the knee. He was skating on artificial limbs. Neither of the assistants said anything. Martinelli thought they were both half in shock.

A few weeks before, Martinelli had decided to tell his wife. At first, Joyce thought he was making a bad joke.

"I'm telling you," said Martinelli.

The next time she saw Andrew skate that was all she could think about. Had it been her, she would have sat in a chair all day and moped, and here was Andrew playing a game most people with two good legs couldn't play. If, God forbid, that had happened to her own son, no way she would have put him on skates. She gave Scott credit for taking the chance. He was a better choice for that job than she.

Once, when Andrew fell and remained down for long seconds, another mother asked Joyce why her husband wasn't taking him off the ice; the boy had obviously hurt his foot or something. Joyce didn't elaborate on it.

Martinelli drove to American Trophy in East Providence. He planned to order a Comeback Player of the Year award. One of the girls there asked whom it was for. A little boy, he explained, who had lost both legs but played hockey. As Martinelli put it, the girl's face "was down to here."

When Martinelli went back to pick up the trophy, the owner came out. Was there really a boy playing hockey with no legs?

Yeah. The kid's amazing, Martinelli said.

The owner took out an etched-glass trophy they had just made for the president of a corporation. He said he wanted to make another for this boy, on the house. Here was Martinelli ordering a thirty-eight-dollar trophy, and the glass one must have been worth four or five hundred dollars.

The hockey banquet was in April of 1999. Five hundred people were expected. Martinelli knew he should be the one to get up there and say something about Andrew, but the idea intimidated him. In his words, Martinelli would rather stick pins in his eyes than talk in front of a crowd. He once turned down being best man so he wouldn't have to give a speech. Then he said to himself, "This kid's got to wake up, deal with this every day of his life. If I can't stand up there for ten minutes, say what I got to say, then something's wrong here."

It was a long banquet. They gave awards to every player, and no one paid much attention except when their own kids were up. It took a few hours to get to Andrew's team. By then you could barely hear the coaches yelling out the names. Martinelli had an assistant coach announce the individual trophies—that was how much he hated speaking in public.

Finally, it was Martinelli's turn. He took the microphone and said he had a special situation. There was something fairly important he wanted to do for one of his kids. That sounded different enough that some people began to quiet down. Martinelli said he had an award for the comeback player of the year. It was usually given to people who return from a possible career-ending injury, but this situation was more intense than that.

"We have a little boy here," Martinelli said, "who, eighteen or twenty months ago, contracted bacterial meningitis."

For a second he wasn't sure he could bring this off, but he kept going.

"He's lucky that he has his life," said Martinelli, "but he didn't pull through it unscathed." By now there was almost total silence. Even the younger kids had mostly stopped talking.

The meningitis, Martinelli said, was very severe, and the boy's doctors had to amputate both his legs. But he came out to play hockey this year. He skated the entire season with two artificial limbs. And no one knew.

At that point, you could have heard a pin drop.

"Andrew Bateson," the coach said, "come on up here." He asked Scott to come up too.

People began to applaud. Andrew walked to the front, turned, and looked back out at everyone. Coach Martinelli put a hand on his head. It was a long time before people stopped clapping. Martinelli gave Andrew the thirty-eight-dollar award, then told about the person at American Trophy who had created a special etched-glass plaque for Andrew. Martinelli showed it to the crowd. It was maybe two feet high. COMEBACK PLAYER OF THE YEAR, it said. It featured two hawks, the symbol of the league. It also had Andrew's name and jersey number, 3.

Martinelli stepped back, leaving Andrew there alone. Everyone in the ballroom was on their feet. Rebecca was supposed to be taking pictures, but she got too emotional. Martinelli didn't see a dry eye in the place. Even the tougher coaches were losing it.

Scott and Andrew went back to their table. The league's mite team, nine-year-olds, had won the state championship. They got pins as the best players in their age group in Rhode Island. One of them came over to Andrew. "I want you to have my championship pin," he said. To Martinelli that said it all. A pin like that means everything to a young kid, and he gives it away. By then you could have mopped the floor with everyone's tears. People kept coming by to shake Andrew's hand and say things like, "You're a heck of a kid."

When the season was still going, Martinelli got a Christmas card from the Batesons showing Andrew in front of the family tree. Inside the card Andrew wrote, *Thanks Coach!* He signed it with his name and jersey number. Martinelli put it on his refrigerator and decided to leave it there. Even a year later, he sometimes got choked up glancing at it. He wished he didn't, but he couldn't help it.

Chapter 17

"We've just gotten into this thing and can't get out . . ."

Rebecca decided that theirs had turned into one of "those" marriages. Scott's anger had diminished, which was a relief, but they weren't at all connected. Rebecca had little interest in trying to fix it. It seemed like too much work. Mostly, they co-existed.

Scott was aware of it too. He felt that he and Rebecca were just sharing the same spot. It was hard for him to imagine them going on like this, but neither could he see leaving; they were still a family.

Jennifer suggested to her sister Rebecca that she and Scott go away for a weekend, no kids.

Rebecca didn't want to force something that might not be there. If they came out of that weekend with nothing, that would be it.

Rebecca found it a bit ironic that she had to spend as much time in shoe stores as before. Whenever they built Andrew a new pair of prosthetics, the feet had to be in scale, which meant new sneakers, new skates, new everything. She pretty much stuck with the self-serve–type shoe stores, so a clerk didn't have to fit him. It was easier not to have to explain the whole thing.

. . .

After waking up, Andrew would begin the process by tightly pulling a thick, silicone sock over the bottom of each leg. The socks had two-inch pins on the ends, pointing straight out. They looked like large screws. Andrew would guide the prostheses over the pins until they clicked into a locking mechanism, the upper shells hugging the silicone. That was how he got his legs on.

In spring of 1999, Andrew developed a severe pressure point near one of his knees. It made it hard to walk. Some days were so bad that Rebecca had to carry Andrew up the stairs at school, though not into his classroom; Andrew insisted on walking that part. It made her realize that he swallowed a lot of pain during the day.

Rebecca told her sister Janice it was taking an hour or more to get Andrew's legs on. That was how tender the sore point had become. The ordeal left Andrew a wreck, Erin late for school, and Rebecca late for work. She didn't know how they would solve this. Janice knew things weren't hunky-dory over there, as she put it. Some families' mornings were about getting Cocoa Puffs for their kids, but not Rebecca's. They tried different silicone covers and consulted another orthopedic surgeon, but nothing worked. It went on for weeks and weeks. Janice felt that Rebecca was as stressed as she had been in some time.

Rebecca made an appointment at Rhode Island Hospital to talk about Andrew's leg pain. She had a handicapped license plate, which she only used when Andrew was having bad days. The last month had been such a time. She drove to the hospital with Andrew and Erin. The closest lot, primarily handicapped spaces, was full. Rebecca noticed that most cars lacked special plates. Many were doctors' cars, which aggravated Rebecca. They'd act differently, she thought, if they faced a single day of what her son had to go through.

Rebecca saw a security officer and waved him down. He asked what the problem was. At that, Rebecca began to lose it. Her son had no legs, she said, and these people had taken all the spaces and didn't care. No one was giving them tickets, or doing anything about it. The officer sympathized. Just put it in the fire lane, he said.

Rebecca wasn't playing that game. Two wrongs, she said, won't make this right. "I'm not parking in the fire lane. What you're going to do is write tickets, and then you're going to help me find a spot." Surprisingly, the security man agreed. He began to put tickets on windshields. It made her feel a little better, but not much.

She went inside for the appointment. The doctor had no clear ideas for Andrew's pain. They could try new silicone covers or tweak the prosthetic shell, but even that would have to wait a few days since his bad leg hurt too much. Erin and Andrew said they had to use the bathroom. That left Rebecca alone with the doctor. She had wanted a quick adjustment so Andrew would be like new, but clearly that wasn't going to happen. The doctor suggested other things to try, but Rebecca was no longer listening closely. She said it wasn't fair. Andrew had fought his way back for two years, and now there was this reversal. She tried to stop herself from crying, but was unable to.

At home that night, Rebecca was back on the parking lot issue. She was thinking of printing flyers saying, PLEASE RESPECT HANDICAPPED RULES. Either that or WERE YOU BORN AN ASS-HOLE? She wasn't the type to use such language, especially on paper, but she was still beside herself. Scott told her it probably wouldn't help.

At least it would make Rebecca feel better.

Scott reminded her that she worked at a church. What would the priests think?

It's not as though she would sign the flyers, she told Scott.

He nodded his head. Rebecca clearly needed to vent.

Andrew's leg problems continued into the summer of 1999. It sometimes left him in a wheelchair or just hanging around the house.

Andrew asked his mom why this had to happen.

"Honey," said Rebecca, "you do so much with your legs, you sometimes get boo-boos." He seldom complained, though. Had it been Rebecca, that's all she would have done. But Andrew didn't get caught up in the whys.

A few times, Andrew did tell his dad he wished he had his old legs.

"Me too," said Scott. "But you're not just your legs. You're a funny kid. You're a cool kid. That's what counts."

Andrew took that in. To Scott, that was about the lowest Andrew seemed to get. It always passed pretty quickly. Scott kept expecting worse. He wasn't sure why it didn't happen.

Once Rebecca was tucking Andrew into bed. It was a warm night and she was barefoot.

"You know, Mom," Andrew said, "I really want to just wiggle my toes."

"Oh really."

She waited for him to say more, but that was it.

"Good night, honey."

"Good night, Mom."

The family went on an apple-picking outing to Barton Farms in the countryside. Rebecca carried Andrew on her back. He had his legs on, but because of the soreness he wasn't able to handle walking. Erin and several cousins had come along. They darted ahead and began to climb trees.

"I'll just sit here," said Andrew.

"All right," said Rebecca. "I'll sit with you."

"I'm sorry, Mommy."

"For what?"

"Because you can't pick apples."

No, Rebecca was sorry that Andrew couldn't.

"Me too," he said.

He picked up a fallen branch and tried knocking apples off the tree above them.

. . .

Even if Andrew didn't seem to get mad about things, Rebecca sometimes did. She got mad at God. *Enough, already,* she thought. *What are you trying to teach Andrew now?* Couldn't God give the bad day to someone else? Andrew was only eight. Hadn't he had his share? Then again, perhaps God was pushing him as a test. And maybe that made him stronger, or at least showed his strength. Theoretically, every day for Andrew could be a bad day, but he didn't let it be, and Rebecca supposed that said something.

That didn't mean Rebecca let God off the hook. Often, she was quite angry at Him.

"Dad," Andrew said, "I want to go outside."

"Andrew, you don't have your legs on." He still couldn't tolerate his prosthetics.

That's okay, said Andrew. He just wanted to see what was going on. Scott prepared to come help, but before he could, Andrew hopped off the couch and propelled himself out the door with his arms. He spotted some kids across the street and called them over. Scott brought out his wheelchair and, next he knew, the kids were pushing Andrew up and down the sidewalk. He ended up sitting on the Mullens' steps. Everyone started doing gymnastics and somersaults. Andrew joined in, without legs. In some ways, he was doing a nimbler job of it. Scott had to give him credit; having his legs off didn't exactly stop him.

Rebecca was outside on College Road, watching the kids. It was getting to be evening. She looked back at her house. It had a nice glow to it. It seemed warm and cozy from where she stood. But it struck her that inside, between her and Scott, things weren't like that. She wished she could get that old sense of security back again. She didn't see how that would be possible.

Father Ken came by. He, Rebecca, and Scott sat on the backyard deck. They talked into the evening. It was the summer of 1999.

Father Ken spoke about some relatives who were having marriage trouble. They had drifted apart and resented each other for it. They were thinking about separating.

To Rebecca, it was almost as if Father Ken was talking about her and Scott.

After he left Scott said, "Sounds a lot like us, doesn't it?"

The comment stunned Rebecca. Until that moment, she wasn't sure Scott was aware of it. In a way, it was unsettling. It made it clear that she wasn't just imagining things. Still, she thought that maybe they would now find a way to talk about it. In all this time they had not yet done so. The comment just hung there, though. Neither followed up on it.

Julie Gatta did not consider it chance that Andrew was assigned to her third-grade class at the Kennedy School. She was twenty-four and tended to see things from a religious perspective. She believed that God often connects us with people we are capable of watching out for; everything had a purpose and reason. She had been a long-term sub at Kennedy the year before and that was supposed to be it, but three days before the 1999 year started, they'd called with an opening. After she accepted, they told her she would have a boy named Andrew Bateson who was a double amputee from meningitis. They said he functioned well in class, but sometimes got bad headaches and had lately been having leg pain. Miss Gatta felt that God had sent her back to Kennedy, believing she had the patience to work with such a child.

Miss Gatta had the kids do a lot of journal writing. Andrew wrote mostly about playing with friends, video games, and family outings. You would not have known his leg situation from his journal; he didn't get into those kinds of details. Miss Gatta didn't think he was hiding anything. He had moved on, that's all.

He was a medium student. Chatty, but otherwise never a problem. He liked gym, computers, art, and reading if it was about sports. To be honest, Miss Gatta thought his handwriting was pretty poor. There were four or five others whose letters were just as poor. All were boys. In Andrew's case, she wasn't sure if there was still a problem with his hands, or if he was a bit lazy.

Miss April was Andrew's CNA again. Because of his leg pain, she had to help a lot more. Miss April knew people who had a little sniffle and did nothing but complain, complain, complain, but that wasn't Andrew. There were times his leg was hurting so badly she would see the redness in his face, but he wouldn't say anything. It was up to Miss April to see when to intervene.

Finally, the parents took Andrew to see Dr. D'Amato, his orthopedic surgeon. Other doctors had diagnosed his pressure points as chronic inflammation. Dr. D'Amato looked deeper. Early on, he had warned the Batesons about bone spurs. When little kids lost a leg, he said, they often developed tiny, spiked growths at the end of the bone, like saw-teeth; it was just a matter of time. It seemed early for that to have happened, and Scott didn't want to believe it, since spurs would require another surgery. But Dr. D'Amato confirmed it; all these months, that had been the problem. Scott and Rebecca hated the idea of doing the operation right after school had started, but maybe Andrew could heal in time for hockey.

The surgery was to be outpatient. Just in case, Rebecca dressed in something she could sleep in. They settled into the pre-op waiting room. Andrew had brought eight games for his Game Boy. He went through each in about two minutes, which Rebecca considered a sign of nerves.

A nurse came in to say it was time. Andrew seemed to be tense. "As soon as you go to sleep," said Rebecca, "your mouth will open and the butterfly will fly out." They wheeled him into the operating room and put a clear mask over his mouth. Rebecca told him it would make him fall asleep. Soon, Andrew's face became a blank stare. It reminded Rebecca of his state in intensive care. She held it together until he was under, then broke down. She was dressed in a yellow hospital johnny, a familiar item.

After a few hours, Dr. D'Amato came out to report his progress. Andrew, he said, had a bursa overlying a sharp spike. He had removed it and trimmed back the bone. There were also some issues on his other leg. Andrew's two lower bones, the tibia and fibula, were diverging. It was called oppositional overgrowth, and could in time be a problem. It was common among child amputees. D'Amato thought they should leave that be for now. It was best not to handicap both sides.

He knew the Batesons expected to go home today but suggested Andrew stay overnight for pain management. That was all Rebecca needed: another night in the hospital.

Andrew went home in a leg cast and after a few days, he could no longer sit still. He started crawling everywhere, the cast making a grating sound against the wood. Rebecca's floors were soon scratched all over.

He returned to school in a wheelchair. Andrew seemed sensitive about it, but his friends got protective. Once Miss Gatta heard one tell a kid from another class, "You shouldn't ask people what's wrong with them." Miss Gatta was impressed with that.

Scott admitted to himself that he had been low for a while. He had never thought to talk about it with anyone, certainly not a counselor. That, he felt, would be selfish—to focus on his own issues instead of Andrew's. But lately he worried that his mood was playing out on both children. As much as Scott tried not to show things in front of the kids, he realized they were likely seeing it anyway.

That would be the worst thing, he felt, for Andrew: to think his illness had caused a problem in his dad, or, worse, between his parents. That would have been a real sin, Scott believed. That could do as much harm to Andrew as losing his legs. Well, perhaps not that much, but enough.

Scott thought: *You're on this earth for what—doctors now give you eighty to eighty-five years?* How much of that time did he want to spend resentful at what had happened? Better to try enjoying life as much as he could. That was certainly what Andrew was doing.

The kids were in and out of the house. Rebecca was cleaning up a downstairs closet. It was a Saturday morning in October of 1999.

Scott was sitting at the kitchen table. He turned to Rebecca and said something about what a nice day it was.

As small a thing as it was, it took Rebecca aback. It was the kind of normal, conversational exchange they hadn't had in some time. It felt different for him to act attentive to her.

Then Scott said, "We've kind of lost something."

The comment came right out of the blue.

Rebecca didn't see any point in reassuring him. She said she agreed. She said things weren't good between them.

She asked, "What can we do about it?" Then she asked if there was anything left to do.

"I don't know," said Scott. What he meant was he didn't know where to start.

"I'm not happy," said Rebecca. "And I can't continue like this."

Scott asked what she thought their options were.

Rebecca told him about that day she was outside, looking at the warm glow of their home and realizing it wasn't like that inside anymore.

Scott stood. Then he took a step toward Rebecca and held her. It had been quite a while since he had done such a thing. "We're going to try to get back to normal," he said.

She stood there with him.

"I know things have been bad," said Scott. "We have to make things better."

He said: "It's not that I don't love you. I don't know what it is. I just have felt . . . not right. Angry, I guess."

Rebecca said, "For the last couple of years, I've been making excuses for why you're angry." She said she had begun to feel this could go on and on. She didn't think she could do that. "It's not fair to me," she said. "It's not fair to the kids."

Scott told her it was nothing Rebecca did, or didn't do. It was just everything that had happened.

For the first time in a while, Rebecca felt some hope. At the same time, she wondered if they still needed something dramatic, some shake-up to push them one way or another.

She asked: "Do you think you should leave?" She expected Scott to lash out at her verbally, to insist there was no way he was leaving his kids. But he answered calmly.

"I don't know if I can go back to my father's," said Scott.

Although she had been the one to ask, it disturbed her that he had already thought about the question.

A part of Rebecca didn't want Scott to move out. She still had a lot of respect for him as a father. But another part of her didn't know anymore. She was struck by her own lack of emotion. She had become kind of numb to the whole thing.

They talked for a long time. They came back to the question of separating. If Rebecca did feel he should move out, said Scott, he would not fight to take the kids with him. This house was where they belonged.

"It's not that I don't love you," said Rebecca. "We've just gotten into this thing and we can't get out of it."

Scott said he knew he had been treating Rebecca as if everything were somehow her fault. That's not what he meant to do. But he could see that's how she might have taken his anger—and distance. Scott told her their marriage was the most important thing. He knew it wouldn't last if he didn't change. He told her he would work hard to keep her.

Rebecca said she just wanted to get back to where they were before Andrew got sick. Scott said he did also. The two decided not to separate.

The hospital had put two stops behind Andrew's wheelchair to keep it from tilting backwards. His parents considered them necessary, as Andrew often tried to do wheelies. Andrew also enjoyed "walking" the chair, muscling it from one wheel to the other so that it moved like a large insect. There was a small set of stairs leading to the back door off the Batesons' kitchen. A few times Andrew asked his mother if he could go down them in the chair, like an extreme-game trick. Rebecca told him absolutely not. He had once done that as a baby in a walker, with a little assistance from his sister.

The Batesons took their kids to the big downtown mall. They paused at the atrium window to see what was going on with the Gravity Games, which NBC was staging in the center of Providence. They happened to see a motorcyclist sail into the air. It was some sight. "Dad," Andrew started saying, "could we go see that? Could we?" Andrew was still in his wheelchair. Outside, they maneuvered over TV cables strung across the ground. The stands were packed, so they stopped in front of a jumbo screen simulcasting the event. Andrew was mesmerized.

"Dad, you see that?" he kept saying.

Yes, Andrew.

"Dad, Dad, that's the kind of dirt bike I want. Really bad."

I know you do, bud.

The motocross riders did midair tricks such as the Superman, where they extended their bodies off the seat while holding the hand grips. Andrew insisted he could do such tricks. Could they get a dirt bike so he could start practicing?

"Dad's not going to buy that for you, Andrew. You're only eight years old." The men on those motorcycles were much older, Scott said. Some were in their thirties. They probably hadn't been allowed to start riding until at least age eighteen. Just then, on the screen, they introduced a rider by saying that no wonder he's so good since he started dirt-biking at six years old. Of course Andrew caught that. He looked at his dad with that "gotcha" smile of his, and said, "See?"

"Andrew," said Scott, "Mom and Dad aren't going to let you ride a bike like that."

Fine, he would ask Santa for it. Rebecca said Santa wasn't likely to bring motorcycles for children. Then she gave Scott a look, like she thought he might fold and had better not. In this case Scott was as firm as she. On the screen, the latest rider soared several stories high. You would have to be crazy, thought Scott, to want to try such a thing.

"I know I can do that," said Andrew.

That December, the Batesons brought Andrew and Erin to see a mall Santa. Afterward, the Santa called Scott and Rebecca aside. He told them Andrew had asked for a dirt motorcycle. The Santa thought Andrew looked a little young for that. How did the parents feel?

Andrew, they said, was indeed too young. Anything the Santa could do to help would be appreciated.

The Santa invited Andrew back. Then he said his rules didn't let him bring motorcycles to children. Andrew appeared a little betrayed. He gave the Santa a once-over.

"Can I ask you a question?" he said.

Yes.

"You the real guy?"

Well, no, the man said. The real Santa hired helpers, and he was one. He asked what gave it away.

The beard, said Andrew. He wasn't buying it.

He got off the man's lap, turned to Rebecca, and said he wanted to see another Santa. Rebecca told him they all followed the same rule book.

In many ways, Andrew gave Miss Gatta perspective on her own life. Before, she would complain about silly things, like needing to lose five pounds. Once she caught herself dwelling on her legs being too fat, then thought about Andrew and realized how stupid that was.

Miss Gatta went to 7 A.M. Mass Mondays and Fridays at St. Sebastian's in Providence. She also went Sundays. Many of her students came from broken homes and she felt they needed prayers. Miss Gatta saw popular culture as fairly gloomy and very much into violence, and prayed that her kids would not get drawn into that. She also prayed that Andrew would have the faith to make it through each day. Miss Gatta worked hard as a teacher, but she believed prayer made the biggest difference in the world.

Chapter 18

"Are you going to say he can't do it?"

The Batesons switched to a new prosthetics shop outside Providence called Next Step. On their first visit, there was a big guy in the waiting area who introduced himself as Jim Donahue. He was wearing long pants, so Rebecca couldn't tell what his situation was. After they took Andrew in, Jim Donahue said he was also a below-knee amputee, both legs.

How did it happen?

He grew up near freight trains, he said. Sometimes his older siblings would jump them for brief rides. He decided to try it, and climbed on okay. Then the train started to speed up. Donahue jumped off, but got his arm caught and fell under the wheels.

Rebecca explained about the meningococcemia.

Donahue said he could see that Andrew was okay with it. He seemed like an exceptional kid. If Rebecca ever had questions, Donahue would be happy to chat.

During a later appointment, the Next Step people told Rebecca a package had been left for Andrew. It was from Jim Donahue. She opened it. There was an old war medal inside. There was also a letter.

"Hi Andrew," it said. "My name is Jim Donahue. We met at Next Step. When I lost my legs in a train accident at four and a half, an old man who was a war veteran came to see me, and told me to be strong and brave in all things I do. Then he gave me this badge of courage, and said I could look at it when things got tough, and draw some strength remembering all the brave people who had it before me. And now I am passing it on for you to use when you need it."

Rebecca decided the medal meant too much just to hand it to Andrew. She called Donahue to ask if he could give it in person. He came for dinner on Memorial Day of 2000. Afterward, Rebecca told Andrew that Mr. Donahue had something for him. She stressed that it meant an awful lot to Mr. Donahue. She didn't want Andrew to be a typical nine-year-old and say "Thanks," then take off.

She had the two sit outdoors on the back deck. Donahue gave him the medal; it was bronze with a ribbon. It said SNOW DRIFT LODGE NO. 246. The ribbon said B. OF R.R. T. CHAPLEAU ONTARIO. He told Andrew about it being a badge of courage.

Rebecca found a place for it in Andrew's bedroom. A few months later, Andrew got really sick with a migraine. He was in a lot of pain. They took him to the emergency room. While there, he said, "Mom, I really need that medal now." That told Rebecca that he understood what it was about.

In spring of 2000, Rebecca took Andrew to be cast for new legs. Andrew said he wanted ones he could both walk and swim in so he didn't have to change them. The Next Step people said it could be done by leaving off the cosmetic coverings. But there was a down-side: the legs would then be alloy rods.

Fine, said Andrew, leave them uncovered.

"You know, honey," Rebecca told him, "it's going to be a lot more obvious." People, she said, might look at him funny.

He didn't care. So they went ahead and made uncovered legs.

To Rebecca, they looked odd: rods attached to two little mini-skis—the feet were to be covered later for shoes. She was unsettled by the sight of them. They reminded her of Inspector Gadget. But Andrew seemed proud of how different the legs were. "Watch, Mom," he said, and began jumping up and down. He got a bit more spring since the ankle bent on this model. It left Rebecca a nervous wreck. It seemed he might just tip over.

When they got home, Andrew headed from house to house to show everyone. Can Alicia come out? Katy? The Days? Rebecca watched from her front steps. The appearance of the legs got to her. Just when she thought she was accepting things, a moment like this—her son walking on rods—whacked her in the face. Still, that was her issue, not his.

On the way to school the next day, Rebecca had a knot in her stomach. Andrew had insisted on shorts, and to her, the new legs made him seem like the bionic boy. She was ready to eyeball anyone who looked at him wrong. A few kids did a double take, but only out of curiosity. They weren't put off by it. Before leaving, Rebecca explained to the principal, Mrs. Koshgarian, that Andrew had new legs that weren't covered, and if anyone said anything, leave them for Rebecca.

At the end of the day, she was told things went fine. The kids thought the legs were pretty cool.

Being out in public with the new legs was different; Andrew got his share of stares. Folks would glance and then whisper to each other. Sometimes Rebecca read their lips. "That's a shame," people said. Rebecca knew it was meant kindly, but she didn't like the "poor thing" response. For his part, Andrew didn't pay much attention to it. Maybe, thought Rebecca, that was the boy in him. He didn't notice a whole lot.

Andrew liked to play outside in bare feet. He thought he could run faster without shoes. Over the weeks those prosthetic feet got beaten up pretty badly. The Batesons tried to keep up with duct tape, but eventually the hard foam began to flop around. They had to replace the foot covers two or three times.

The hospital had a program with Shake-A-Leg that taught sailing to kids with disabilities. Andrew signed up for it. They headed out on the bay from Newport. Andrew's former social worker, Robin Vargas, was along as a hospital staffer. She ended up on the same boat as Andrew. It was a perfect, sunny day. Pretty soon it was Andrew's turn at the tiller. Robin watched him steer the boat, his brown hair in the wind and a big grin on his face. She thought back to those early days when he was in a coma. It was one of the nicer moments she could recall professionally.

Before the sailing camp, Andrew had again needed his prosthetic feet re-covered. The technician misunderstood and covered the whole legs. Andrew didn't like that one bit, preferring the nimbler freedom of the rods. Rebecca told him it wasn't the end of the world. While sailing, the foam covers absorbed water, and two days later Andrew was still leaving puddles around the house. They also found that seawater didn't age well in spongy material. They had to take the legs back to be uncovered again. The people at Next Step told them Andrew was quite an unusual case.

Occasionally Andrew got invited to birthday parties where he knew only one or two kids. Had Scott had prosthetic legs, he would have been uncomfortable among new people, but Andrew was up for anything. He never hesitated. He sometimes became the center of attention at such events—when, for example, the other boys asked him to burp their names, a talent Andrew wasn't shy about. His parents were less than thrilled.

Andrew was climbing a slide at a playground when a younger boy grabbed one of his legs and began pulling it. He would not let go. Andrew decided to release it, and the leg popped off right into the boy. It bumped near his eye. The boy was too surprised to cry; he just handed it back. Rebecca was sitting across the way with Scott and thought she saw one of Andrew's prosthetics go flying. As she was asking Scott to investigate, a child from the block came over and told them what had happened. Rebecca had to admit she got a kick out of the way Andrew responded. Releasing the leg probably beat yelling or fighting. Andrew didn't bother to mention it until his parents asked.

Cindy Day, the Batesons' neighbor, had doubted that Andrew would fit easily back into the pace of the block. In terms of sports and such, there was only so much one could expect, she thought. A year after Andrew got out of the hospital, Cindy no longer felt that way. Andrew was particularly good on a bicycle. Sometimes the kids had races. As he pedaled, Andrew often looked around to see where the others were; his whole focus was winning. At one point, they went through a phase of rear-ending each other for fun. The idea was to slam to a stop just inches from the bike in front of you. Andrew loved that game, especially when people misjudged. When the kids played it, Mike Day noticed that Rebecca never looked.

Cindy had long thought Andrew had an issue with limits. When he was younger, Rebecca never let go of his hand in parking lots. When they went to pools, he'd jump in before Rebecca told him it was okay. He wasn't the kind to pause and think, *What if?* Soon after the hospital, Cindy noticed the same tendency. It wasn't enough for him just to ride his motorized three-wheeler, he had to stand on it. Later, he resumed skateboarding down driveways into the street, although he was told not to. Cindy Day thought he had not changed much.

Andrew talked his dad into constructing a ramp so he could practice bicycle jumps. Scott assured Rebecca it would be fine, it was only four inches at the high end. Still, she considered it a bad idea.

"Rebecca," Scott said, "are you going to say he can't do it?"

As a matter of fact, she said, yes.

"Then you come up with a reason to tell him."

Rebecca was not laughing about this. She told Scott he was on his own. "When he breaks his arm," she said, "you take him to the emergency room and explain why you let a bilateral amputee child do that." Soon Andrew was catching air. By then, Rebecca had gone back into the house. Sometimes she wasn't at all amused by Scott and Andrew's choice of games.

When Scott was at work, Andrew asked Rebecca to set up the ramp. At first she said no. Then she remembered what her mother-in-law used to say about not breaking Andrew's spirit. When he would overdo things, Agnes Bateson said it wasn't bad behavior, it was his personality, and it shouldn't be bottled up. Rebecca knew she was right. She agreed to take out the bike ramp, but this was the hardest area for her as a mom of an amputee: not standing in his way.

Long before Andrew got sick, Agnes used to turn to her husband and say, "Who does Andrew remind you of?" Jim would point to Scott and answer, "Right there. The father."

Jim and Agnes Bateson had five children, four of them boys. Scott got into the most mischief. Once, while grocery shopping with the kids, the parents heard a big crash. Agnes asked what it might be. "I think I know," said Jim. He was right. Scott had knocked over a stack of cans.

Another time the family went to Slater Park on Easter. They strolled past a fountain. Jim Bateson turned to see Scott wading in the water with his older brother Jimmy. They were still wearing their new shoes and Easter suits.

Andrew liked to hear these stories. "Poppy," he asked his grandfather, "was my father always getting into trouble?"

"Oh, yes," said Jim. "Just like you, Andrew." He meant it.

Jim Bateson never scolded Andrew for going too fast or too hard. He just thought to himself, *God bless him.* He didn't think he should be on Andrew's back, saying "Don't do this" and "Don't do that." If Andrew wasn't afraid of things, why talk him into it? Jim got that outlook from his wife, Agnes. As Andrew's dad, Scott had the same outlook. Even Rebecca was coming around to it. Well, sometimes. Jim guessed that went a long way toward explaining why Andrew seemed to cope so well.

...

Rebecca phoned her sister Jen to see how Andrew was doing; he had gone to Jen's house for a sleepover with his cousins. Jen always got a kick out of having Andrew over. You never knew what would come out of his mouth. He once told her that when he got married, he would pick a woman without legs.

Jen mentioned that he had been hanging out with his prosthetics off. Rebecca said he at least had to put the tight silicon covers on to keep the skin desensitized. Jen relayed the message. Rebecca heard Andrew say, "I'll do it for five bucks." Jen made a counteroffer to her nephew. How about a dollar?

"Don't you dare pay him," Rebecca told her sister.

Jen was enjoying her moment of influence. "This is my house," she said. "We can do whatever we want at my house."

In the end, Andrew got her up to three dollars. Jen respected how good he was at manipulating her. He really knew how to work the system.

The aunts liked to trade Andrew stories. One winter day, while at Deb's house, he came in from playing and took off his shoes. Deb told him he needn't bother.

"My feet are cold," he said.

It took her a moment.

Rebecca was surprised at how easily Andrew joked about his legs and feet. When closing car doors, she always said, "Watch out for hands and feet." Andrew would respond to the feet part with, "Come on, Mom."

Every so often, if someone stepped on his foot, he acted like it hurt, just to mess with the person.

Scott's brother was having his fiftieth birthday at a restaurant banquet room. They had a DJ there named Smilin' Sam who pulled silly things out of a bag—a rubber chicken, ladies' underwear—and asked if someone had lost this. Then he pulled out a fake leg. Scott was taken aback. The DJ asked if it belonged to anyone. At that,

Andrew walked toward the stage, took off a leg, and held it up. He pointed to the one in the DJ's hand and said he thought that might be his other one. The DJ was stunned. Andrew then put his leg back on. Scott was struck by how little self-consciousness Andrew had. Not that Scott minded. It certainly was better than Andrew being in a shell.

The Batesons were at the home of the Amarals. The kids were quite hyper, Andrew more so than the others. He began playing a keyboard loudly, and Rebecca told him to turn it off.

"Come on," Andrew said, "one more song."

"Andrew," Rebecca said loudly.

"Just one."

Maria could see he was driving Rebecca a little nuts.

Andrew!

There was a time when Rebecca thought he would never live to the point where she would be yelling at him again.

A half dozen kids from College Road sat on Andrew's front steps. Most were girls. The block happened to have more of them. They were between the ages of eight and thirteen. Stephanie Day from across the street said things weren't the same when Andrew was in the hospital. It was boring, added Alicia Mullen; hardly any laughs. Andrew was the one who made things on the block fun. Amanda Day said they were like a circle, and if one part was missing, it didn't work.

One of them pointed a few inches below Andrew's knee.

"About right here," she said.

"Show him," said another.

Andrew pushed the release button and removed his leg. The others said they weren't freaked out by it. If Andrew could handle it, they could. Then they said they had a performance to demonstrate. They gathered on a lawn and linked arms, Andrew in the middle. One of them pushed Play on a boom box and, somewhat in tune, they began to sing, "Keep smiling. Keep shining. Know you can always count on me, for sure. That's what friends are for . . ." Then the CD skipped and they said they had to start over. Next they did a Backstreet Boys song. They sang, "If you want it to be good, girl, get yourself a bad boy." Andrew, they explained, was playing that part.

They sat on the stairs again. Several remembered the night he got sick. "The next morning," said Alicia Mullen, "he had purple spots." Then he was in a coma. Alicia said everyone thought he was going to die.

Andrew was asked why he didn't get depressed. Amanda whispered something to him.

"I have my friends," he said.

"Sometimes," Brianne Day said, "I even forget that he had meningitis and his legs were cut off." They said they saw Andrew as the same crazy kid.

Andrew sat in his room, showing it off to a visitor. He was asked what he had in here. "Stars," said Andrew. "They glow in the dark."

What else?

"Electronic skeet shooting."

What was that football?

"Signed."

He had a banner for the local hockey team, the Providence Bruins, and was wearing his Harley vest.

What did he want to be one day?

"A doctor. So I can help everybody." Or maybe a hockey player.

He was chewing gum. He took out some photographs.

"This is me in the hospital. That's Muhammad Ali."

Did he know who that was?

"A wrestler, I think," said Andrew. "I didn't see him 'cause I was sleeping."

He blew a bubble. Another photo showed Andrew with dark circles under his eyes and a nasogastric tube. A large man in motorcycle clothing was standing next to him.

"These are the Harley guys," he explained.

What would Andrew tell other kids if they had the same thing happen to them?

"I don't know."

Did he have a favorite sport?

"Hockey."

A favorite hobby?

"Video games."

Food?

"Chocolate. Like a Hershey bar."

Favorite TV show?

"*Rugrats. Doug.*"

Books?

He lifted a handful of Goosebumps titles from a shelf.

"I already read all these, but I forgot to read this one."

A bit later, he sat with his parents downstairs.

"The only thing I can't do like when I was regular," he said, "is run as fast."

But he could jump better, he said. When he goes to get his stuff from his school closet, he jumps over the other coats so he doesn't have to step on them. He couldn't do that before.

What else can he do better?

He can put his knees behind his head. Watch . . .

On another day, Andrew was standing in the kitchen with Rollerblades on. "I asked for V8 Splash," he told his mother.

"You asked for milk," said Rebecca.

"V8 Splash."

Three other kids were in the den. It was the sort of house where it seemed there were always three other kids around. There was also a beagle-sized mutt named Chrissy who snapped at flies even in winter when none were there, and a cat named Sneakers who originally, said Rebecca, was a girl, but was now an it.

Andrew asked why he was picked to be written about.

Because even though he had fake legs, he played hockey and bladed and biked.

"And I do ramps," he added.

His family had recently gone to a Providence Bruins game. They had seats on the glass. It was the first professional hockey game Rebecca had been to.

"My mom got freaked out," said Andrew.

"Why?"

"They kept banging against the boards," he said of the players. Whenever they did so, she screamed. It was embarrassing.

At that, he bladed into the den to resume a movie.

"That concludes your interview with Andrew," said Rebecca.

Five minutes later, he rolled back and began asking about the laptop computer a visitor had brought.

"You got a printer for that?" he said. You got a case for it? How many laptops you got? You got one at work?

He then rolled out of the kitchen. He seldom stopped moving.

Later, Andrew went outside to play roller hockey in a neighbor's driveway. Most of the players were the girls he had sat on the steps with. Andrew was the only one seeming to take it seriously. The other team was winning; with each opposing goal, he got more upset. Pretty soon he worked up to tears. He had a hard time losing.

On another visit Andrew was in the backyard, having camped out overnight in a tent with his sister. He awoke about 10 A.M. Rebecca carried him into the kitchen, where he announced he wanted to go swimming. He had a brief breakfast and spent the rest of the morning in and out of the Batesons' above-ground pool.

Dr. Richard Greco, one of Andrew's pediatricians, continued to see him for regular checkups. Greco noticed that when Andrew had jeans on, it was impossible to tell that there was anything unusual about him. He climbed around the waiting area like any other kid.

In the exam room, Rebecca mentioned that Andrew was in an ice-hockey league.

Greco thought that was one for the books. It got him remembering a hospital discharge meeting he had attended just before Andrew left. One of the physical therapists predicted that within a year or two, Andrew might be doing many things a normal child would. Greco had thought she was living in a fantasy world.

Karen Zelano, family friend and Hasbro nurse, held a party for the Batesons at her house, a potluck dinner. She invited hospital staffers, including Michele Rozenberg, one of the PICU nurses. Mid-evening, Michele glanced into the den and saw Andrew watching TV with the other kids. She was struck by the way he didn't stand out. Michele doubted that Andrew remembered her, which was fine. It was all right with her if the role she played in his life was forgotten.

Ginger Manzo, the psychiatrist, bumped into the Batesons in one of those mall stores full of high-tech gadgets. Scott and Andrew were taking turns trying out a massage chair.

Scott told her Andrew was doing well. "I can't even keep up with him," he said.

Manzo had been unable to get the parents to work on their own issues in counseling. She had worried about that. But Scott and Rebecca seemed connected. It told her you don't always have to do things the way you planned as a treatment provider.

Andrew said a brief hello to Dr. Manzo, but was too busy with various gadgets to have time for her.

Mary St. Jacques, the emergency-room nurse, had a theory as to why Andrew had survived. Partly, it was his personality; he was pretty tenacious. In her experience patients with a strong will had a better chance at a good outcome. As far as everyone praying for him, she thought that was a factor too. There was no way to prove it, but she believed prayer did help.

Karen Zelano did too. On the other hand, Karen had seen children with a lot of prayer who didn't survive. In the end, she felt it was hard to say.

Father Ken Letoile moved on from St. Pius to a new assignment in Cincinnati. They had wanted to transfer him while Andrew was in the hospital, but he asked that it be put off. Father Ken thought St. Pius became a closer church after the healing service held before the operation that had saved Andrew's knees. It was a turning point in people's journey to Christ. It wasn't Scripture that did that; it was this little boy. Father Ken saw a biblical dimension to it: God working through a child to bring a community together. The experience changed Father Ken himself. He had vivid memories of his visits to the pediatric ICU. He experienced a grace there that he guessed people felt when in Jesus's literal presence. Through Andrew, Father Ken had found an intimacy with Christ he considered a singular episode in his priesthood.

Nationally, there are fifteen to twenty localized outbreaks of bacterial meningitis a year, usually involving three to twelve people each. Altogether, there are 3,000 cases reported in America every twelve months. The world's largest outbreaks are in sub-Saharan Africa, where up to 200,000 people have been affected in a year, with 20,000 dying.

The February after Andrew got sick, there had already been eight cases of bacterial meningitis in Rhode Island in two months. At that rate, there would be fifty by year's end, five times the average amount. It was the third straight year with abnormally high clusters.

The state's health director and governor consulted with the Centers for Disease Control in Atlanta, which agreed that something was happening in Rhode Island. Together, they decided to vaccinate all residents between the ages of two and twenty-two—over 250,000 people. It was thought to be the most widespread bacterial meningitis vaccination ever accomplished in the United States.

After it was done, the rest of 1998 saw only four more cases, making a total of twelve, which was about average. The state had only nine cases in each of the next two years. The statewide vaccination apparently worked. At last, the outbreak seemed to be over.

In early 2005, the CDC began recommending a new meningitis vaccine for all college freshmen entering dorms, since the disease can spread through close-quarter living. The vaccine is also suggested for all eleven- and twelve-year-olds. Unlike the old vaccine, which protected for two to five years, the new one is effective for eight years, and tends to kill dormant bacteria in the throats of carriers. It does not cover the B strain, which Andrew got, and which causes almost a third of all cases.

Kevin Sullivan finished his overnight shift at Hasbro's pediatric intensive care unit. It was 8 A.M. He stopped home to change, then drove to a nearby high school, one of many sites for the statewide vaccination. Sullivan began giving injections at 9:30 and by 3 P.M. had finished hundreds. He could not remember the last time he volunteered six hours for anything, let alone after a twelve-hour shift. As he worked, he thought back to Andrew, especially those dressing changes. He continued giving vaccinations until it was done.

Chapter 19

"I got to ride my bike, see ya . . ."

Joseph Mullen was sitting on his front steps with Scott. Mullen tended to be quite spiritual, at least by his own thinking. He always carried a finger rosary with him. It helped him feel wired to God.

"Scott," he said, "you're going to take this one of two ways: that I'm an enlightened individual, or that I'm a freaking nut." Then he said that Andrew was chosen for this. If you had to pick a person to get this disease, he told Scott, it would be the Andrew Bateson type of nature, because he was strong and able to take what came his way. And also that he had a purpose. We're each predestined for certain things, said Mullen. You can bet, he went on, that while in the hospital Jesus Christ and the Blessed Mother and everybody were right there with him. That's why he was healed. And instead of clamming up, Andrew was running with it, inspiring folks, growing as a soul. Look at his hockey. God breathes through all of us, said Mullen.

Scott took that in. He thought that *picked* might not be the right word, but when folks saw Andrew doing his stuff, it did make them rethink their problems. At least that's what some people told him. He didn't say this to Mullen, though. He just sat there quietly.

Mullen smiled to himself, thinking, *He probably thinks I'm a freaking nut.* It didn't bother him. Mullen believed he was right. Had Andrew gotten to the hospital a few minutes later, that would have been it. If that wasn't God, Mullen didn't know what was. Not that Andrew wasn't human. Sometimes Mullen saw him sitting over there with a pensive look. Mullen could imagine his thoughts. It didn't happen often.

There were things Scott still found hard to talk about. Andrew's surgery day, for example. Each anniversary of it, July 22, remained difficult for him.

Once Scott began to pace as he described to someone the time he was told Andrew would lose his legs. He seemed to relive the moment. His voice got loud as he talked of the anger at God he felt that day. Finally, he sat down. "You'd think you could put these things away after a few years," he said.

Sometimes Scott couldn't help but think, *Too bad it happened.* Then he'd start to dwell on it. He didn't share that with anyone, though, not even Rebecca. If someone was going to obsess on such thoughts, just as well that it be Scott.

Early on, the one thing the Batesons thought for sure was that Andrew would be a depressed child. Neither Scott nor Rebecca understood why he wasn't. Scott thought that Andrew was hardly a boy you could ask. If you said, "Where do you get your persistence?" his answer would be, "I don't know. I got to ride my bike—see ya." Scott doubted that Andrew had talked himself into putting this behind him. He didn't think that way. He was just on to the next activity. Scott thought that explained most of it.

One day someone asked Rebecca about Andrew's legs, and she caught herself thinking, *Right, his legs.* It said a lot about Andrew that she wasn't aware of them constantly.

Rebecca believed that Andrew had probably been touched. She suspected that God had given him a little extra. Sometimes she thanked Him for keeping Andrew the same little boy he was before.

It wasn't only God, though; it was also Andrew's friends. That had been Rebecca's greatest fear: how the kids from his block and class might react. But they took him right back in. She thought that was a big part of his recovery. Then again, she wondered whether God had a hand in that, too.

Scott sometimes felt that he and Rebecca were more wounded than Andrew by what happened. Kind of ironic, he thought, that their son, by how he handled it, helped his parents heal. It should have worked the other way.

It did change Rebecca in one sense. She seldom let things get to her the way she used to. If Andrew could cope with what was on his plate, she could too. Except when people parked in handicapped spots. That was one thing that still sent her right over.

Rebecca was constantly watching Andrew for lasting effects of the disease. It took three years for his appetite to come back to where it had been, but it did. Even then, he got thirsty quickly.

In the cold, Andrew wore gloves more readily than other kids. In a pool, his fingertips got numb after a while. Those seemed the only signs of hand damage.

Scott expected Andrew's running to get much faster in the future, especially with better prosthetics. Some of the top designs included advanced shock absorption and hydraulics, which gave better spring to the stride. Most of that technology, however, was for adults, and those models cost through the roof. Many with such prosthetics competed athletically, and were sponsored. Scott understood the economics of it. Maybe in time.

Scott held on to one of the cloth scapulars they had placed below Andrew's knees during his coma. It had a prayer on one side and a picture of the Virgin Mary on the other. Every night Scott put it on his bureau so he could grab it as he left for work. He kept it in his pocket, just to have it with him. Over time he stopped doing that, but it took several years.

Andrew went to tryouts for the 1999 Edgewood Hockey house league. At the time, he still had leg pain from bone-spur surgery, and the drills weren't coming together for him. He had to rest a lot to take the pressure off, and had trouble standing after falls. After a while he gave up and sat on the bench. A coach who knew about Andrew's legs skated over. He saw that Andrew had been crying. The coach asked him what the problem was. Andrew didn't say much. At that point, the coach gave him a talking-to. Did Andrew think pro hockey players never got injured? That Gretzky never got hurt? Bobby Orr? Happened all the time, but they came back strong. "You're on the team," he said, and skated away. Andrew settled in after that. Scott felt it was Andrew's best season.

Scott called his older brother Jimmy. Andrew had a hockey game at Providence College and wanted his uncle there. Once play started, Jimmy couldn't get over it. Andrew was really whizzing after that puck. He took a spill, got up, and went right back into it.

Jimmy looked at his brother. "He's going real good," said Jimmy. "You can't complain about that, Scott."

"Yeah," Scott said. "I know."

For a while there, Jimmy had worried about Scott as much as Andrew, maybe more so. Lately, he thought Scott was finally getting okay with things.

On another day, Andrew's grandfather Jim watched him riding his bicycle. Andrew was really moving. Jim asked Scott if he wasn't afraid for his son.

Scott just said, "Oh, Dad." It made Jim Bateson think back to how distraught Scott had been in the hospital. Scott was different now.

Karen Lamberton, Scott's sister, brought her family to have dinner with the Batesons at the New Buffet restaurant. There were eleven of them there. Andrew took a few bites, got up, and went back for more. So did the other kids. They were constantly back at that buffet. Karen finally said enough was enough, sit down for goodness' sake.

As they were leaving, the kids began running around outside the exit door. Andrew had on shorts, so you could see his prosthetic legs with their alloy rods. A car pulled up near the kids and the driver rolled down the window. It was a black woman. She had a big smile. "God bless you, child," she said. Andrew barely stopped to acknowledge it, which made the woman smile even more. John Lamberton thought, *He's just the way he was before.*

The family drove to Waterville Valley for a weekend of skiing. It was the winter of 2000, Andrew's first time since he lost his legs. He said he was psyched because his feet wouldn't get cold. That kind of humor sometimes threw Scott and Rebecca.

Andrew had gone skiing once before, at age five, a nerve-racking experience for his parents. Rebecca remembered how Andrew had headed straight downhill the moment he got off the first chair. She yelled for him to stop, fall, do something. He just kept going. They warned him not to do that again, but on a later run he did. Rebecca skied after him. When he began to veer toward a ski-school building, she grabbed his hood. He got so frustrated he went limp. That pulled Rebecca down with him, and the two tumbled together. One of her skis cracked his goggles. He was furious. One thing Andrew didn't like was being stopped.

Rebecca assumed he would be less reckless on this trip. They arrived mid-evening and decided to go inner-tube sledding. After the first run Andrew tried walking back uphill, but he didn't get far. Scott and Rebecca had to pull him in the tube. It was a lot of work. A couple times Rebecca could barely catch her breath. Andrew wanted to go again and again.

He woke up with a sore spot near his knee. That usually kept him off his legs for days. The parents spent a half hour getting his prosthetics on. Rebecca did not think it would work, but Andrew made himself take some steps. That was how badly he wanted to ski.

They had to carry him part of the way to the adaptive-ski-school office. There the Batesons explained about his situation and his knee pain. Rebecca said she wasn't sure her son could ski today. Andrew interrupted. He said his leg felt fine. The instructors looked at the parents as if to say, *Get your stories straight, will you?*

Liz Craveiro was the supervisor of Waterville Valley's adaptive program. She was forty-five and an adaptive skier herself, having gotten polio at age three. Her right leg was partly paralyzed, so Liz was a three-track skier. She used one leg and two outriggers, special crutches with ski tips. Although in charge of sixty volunteer instructors, Liz decided to take Andrew herself, in part because they seldom got bilateral amputees. Truth be told, she also thought Andrew might be a kick. He looked like he had that little devil in him. She brought another instructor with her, so it was two on one.

Liz took Andrew to the top of Courtyard, a beginner slope, and tried to teach him to sidestep. Andrew was not paying much attention. He kept looking down the slope. She told him to glide sideways—slowly—with his skis in a wedge. Instead, he pointed straight down and took off. He then fell.

Generally, Andrew was a quick learner, although he didn't really listen when told to traverse. He wasn't interested in tracking slowly side to side. He preferred speed to turning. Liz understood. The feeling of that wind rushing by your face was a freedom that adaptive skiers didn't get in everyday life. Andrew liked being able to go as fast as others. Liz spent a lot of time insisting he traverse. He would do it for half the slope, then shoot downhill. He appeared unable not to.

Rebecca exhaled when Andrew first skied away with the instructors. On such trips it was no picnic being his mother. It was a relief to sign off and let someone else worry about him for a while. She did look for Andrew from the chairlift, however. The first time she saw his jacket she thought it couldn't be him, since he was parallel-skiing. But it was. He had apparently skipped the snowplow.

Andrew noticed other skiers on snow bikes—bicycle frames with skis where wheels would be. Riders clipped mini skis to their boots and rode down that way, turning with handlebars or by leaning. Andrew kept asking if he could try one. Liz Craveiro decided she didn't have much choice. Scott and Rebecca spotted them at that point, and rode up the chair to watch. At the top, Liz told Andrew he could under no circumstances ride a ski bike straight down. They were much faster than skis, so he had to keep turning. As Liz was in mid-sentence, Andrew took off. She went after him. "Turn!" she called out. "Andrew, turn!"

Rebecca was watching this. Liz, she realized, was having a Rebecca-day: Stop. Slow down. Don't.

Andrew was going so fast Liz couldn't catch him. She kept yelling for him to turn, but he didn't. She began to get panicky, since there were chairlift towers on the slope. She had never seen a first-time rider go so fast. By now he had lost control and was tracking toward one of the towers. She was convinced he would hit it. At the last moment, he turned and fell, cartwheeling with the bike. Liz caught up to him.

"I'm okay," he said.

Once she determined that was true, she lost her temper a bit.

"If you ever do that again," Liz said, "you're off the mountain the rest of the day." Liz had spent five years teaching at Waterville's program, and before that, eight years at Loon Mountain. As far as threatening to pull an adaptive skier off the slopes, this was a first. It wasn't her style. She was quite a patient person.

They went on with their lesson. Andrew still resisted turning, but Liz thought they had a blast. Other instructors noticed Andrew, and afterward asked Liz what his disability was. When she told them, they were blown away. After 4 P.M., Liz was in the adaptive ski office filling out her whiteboard for the next day. Three instructors were around. They asked who would be assigned Andrew Bateson; each wanted to take him. That was the first time Liz had instructors bid for a kid they hadn't yet taught. She decided to give him to a young woman named B.J. whose energy level was off the charts. At the end of her lesson with him, B.J. came in saying that Andrew had about worn her out. He wouldn't stop.

Ever since they'd talked about their marriage, Rebecca thought Scott had been really trying. That meant a lot to her. A part of her thought it would last only so long, but the other shoe didn't drop. Gradually she began to trust Scott again. At the end of 2000, she became pregnant with their third child. They had a little girl. They named her Abigail Faith Bateson.

Andrew's kidneys, which failed while he was in the hospital, seemed to recover fully. His skin still had scars from the purpura lesions, but he didn't need grafts, as do some meningococcemia patients.

Early in 2001, Andrew's left leg showed a slight deformity. The fibula, the small lower leg bone, was beginning to hook at the end, in part because Andrew's growth plates were damaged by the disease.

On February 13 of that year, he went for surgery. Dr. D'Amato shaved off the bowed end of the fibula. Then he removed the entire bone, flipped it, and inserted it into the larger tibia, creating one, double-strength unit. The fibula's smooth top end was now at the bottom. D'Amato told the Batesons this would likely end the need for future surgeries and would keep the leg strong enough for prosthetics as Andrew grew.

The recovery was rough. Andrew lost a lot of blood and developed pneumonia. He was in the hospital six days. He was angry that he missed his year-end hockey playoffs and a planned ski trip.

He got the cast off in late April of 2001. A week or so after that, he joined a summer roller-hockey league. He wore long pants to his first practice and, afterwards, his new coach was shocked when Scott told him about Andrew's legs. They kept it quiet, and none of

his teammates seemed to realize his situation. He took his share of
spills on the outdoor concrete rink.

That winter, he switched to a new ice-hockey league. He signed
up again for the 2002–2003 season. By this time, Scott figured it
would be no big deal to tell if it came up. It never did.

The date came for the wedding of Andrew's cousin Bethany. It
was the first one in the family for that generation. The ceremony
was held July 18. Andrew was ring bearer, though he misheard it as
"ring-burier," and at first thought that was his function. A year before, he had still been in a coma. That was when Bethany had said
he would dance at her wedding. The bridesmaids came down the
aisle, then the ushers, and then it was Andrew's turn. He was
dressed in a little tux. As he walked, Rebecca was picturing herself
in yellow scrubs by his hospital bed. So was Scott. The two had a
hard time holding it together. It seemed that others did too. A lot
of people thought Andrew stole the show from the bride. The bride
herself admitted as much. After the ceremony, Rebecca gave him a
big hug, but Andrew shrugged uncomfortably, as if to say, *Don't
embarrass me in front of the guys.*

At the reception, the bride asked if Rebecca and Andrew would
open the dance floor. She even planned a special song, "I Believe I
Can Fly." The two began. By now Andrew's white shirt was untucked and he was missing his bow tie. Half the place was choked
up, watching mother and son whisper to each other as they danced.
They seemed to be having a real heart-to-heart. Most presumed
they were discussing what a triumphant moment this was. In fact,
Andrew was repeatedly asking, "Can we get off now?" He was one
relieved kid when it was over.

Dr. Kleinman moved on from Hasbro to become an intensive-care
attending at Boston Children's Hospital. It was a big change, as she
had been in Providence since medical school. Soon after, she and
her husband had the little boy she had carried while treating Andrew.

From time to time, Kleinman came across new therapies for meningococcemia, but there was nothing revolutionary. Still, she was always looking for better weapons. Her main hope was for a solid, lasting vaccine that could be given to all infants. She thought it was likely to happen in the next twenty years.

Dr. Kleinman tended to see most diseases with a neutral, scientific eye, but this was one she disliked very much. She felt it was hard not to.

Kleinman and her young son, David, came down to Providence to spend the day with the Batesons. Soon after they arrived, Andrew wanted to show her his in-line skating skills. Rebecca, who was about to put lunch on the table, asked Andrew if it had to be now. By that time, he had his helmet on and was out the door. Later, he was out there again on his bike. In Dr. Kleinman's eyes, Andrew had come back to an even greater point than she had considered possible. She took a photograph of him on Rollerblades. Later, she put the picture up in her office at Boston Children's. She often looked at it to remind herself why she does what she does.

Rebecca was asked to give a speech as part of a regional conference on medical trauma. Most of the talks were technical, the audience being hospital people. Her role was to give the perspective of a patient's family. She was supposed to talk for fifteen minutes or so. She thought hard about how to end the speech. Then her mind went to a particular moment.

It had taken place a few months after they had gotten home from the hospital. The Batesons sat down to dinner at the kitchen table. They said grace. As they began to eat, Andrew said, "I saw God, Mommy."

Rebecca sort of caught her breath. She asked Andrew when that had happened.

"When I was sleeping in the hospital."

"You did?"

"Yes. He put His arms out, and I thought He was going to give me a hug, but instead, He just touched me on the shoulder."

For a child to verbalize it that way strengthened what Rebecca had long felt. Perhaps God had changed His mind. She sat there at the table and did not say anything. Andrew just went back to his dinner.

Acknowledgments

I heard about a little boy who lost two legs but now plays ice hockey and decided to write a column about it for my newspaper, the *Providence Journal*. I called Rebecca Bateson, the boy's mother, and came by for an interview.

The family's ordeal had spanned a couple of years, but after a long session, Rebecca and I had barely covered the first half hour. So, instead of a column, I decided to write an in-depth feature. Following a second interview, I realized the story was bigger still. I ended up spending the next year working on a six-part newspaper series.

I lost count of how many times I interviewed Rebecca and her husband, Scott. We met weekends, evenings, and during their lunch breaks. They were both gifted at remembering anecdotes and emotions. This is their story, and more than I, it is they who told it well.

There are few people busier than the attending physician of an intensive-care unit. Dr. Monica Kleinman had that title while treating Andrew, and she later moved to a demanding job at Boston Children's Hospital. Despite that, she gave me many hours for many interviews. I'm in her debt.

There isn't space here to thank everyone else who gave me time; there were dozens. Their names are throughout the book, and I'm grateful to every one of them.

I talked to many agents about helping me with the manuscript. The one who believed in it most was Andy Zack. He proved more than a business adviser. On every level, he was and is a true partner.

I want to thank the people at Center Street, particularly Gary Terashita, my editor. I'll always be grateful for not just the resources at the Time Warner Book Group but, more important, the personal attention.

There's a reason this book found its beginnings as a series in the *Providence Journal:* The paper encourages literary journalism. That comes from the philosophy of the top editor, Joel Rawson; the publisher, Howard Sutton; and editors down through the ranks. I'm particularly grateful to Joel for helping shape the early version of this story.

Finally, for doing the most important work during the many hours I spent on this, my greatest gratitude goes to my wife.